The Autism Diet Guide: A Parent's Path To Improved Behavior And Well-Being

Understanding Food Sensitivities, Implementing a GFCF Diet, Practical Strategies, And Adapt Traditional Flavors To Empower Your Child's Behavioral and Cognitive Health

Tiina Hoddy

Table Of Contents

Foreword

As parents, we're always searching for the best ways to support and nurture our children's growth, happiness, and well-being. For parents of autistic children, this journey often involves additional layers of discovery, seeking out unique strategies and solutions to support the many facets of their development. One of the most impa

ctful, yet often overlooked, approaches is dietary intervention.

"The Autism Diet Guide: A Parent's Path To Improved Behavior And Well-Being" is not just a book; it's a guide born out of compassion, research, and the drive to create positive change in the lives of children and their families. With growing evidence linking nutrition to behavioral and cognitive health, the information compiled here serves as a lifeline for parents who have witnessed firsthand the challenges associated with food sensitivities and dietary triggers in their children.

The goal of this book is not to offer a one-size-fits-all approach but rather to empower parents with knowledge and tools that can be adapted to their unique family circumstances. Within these pages, you'll find a blend of scientific insight, practical advice, and empathetic guidance that makes the sometimes daunting process of dietary change approachable and achievable. Each chapter is thoughtfully structured to take you step-by-step through understanding food sensitivities, implementing a diet that suits your child's needs, and navigating the real-life challenges that come with dietary shifts—all while celebrating every small victory along the way.

As you read through this guide, you will discover that these dietary changes are not merely about removing certain foods but about introducing a pathway toward better health, improved behavior, and a more harmonious family life. The tips and strategies outlined will help you move beyond common obstacles, such as picky eating or navigating social gatherings, with practical solutions and encouragement.

The profound effect that diet can have on an autistic child's well-being is undeniable, but more importantly, this book is a reminder that every step forward is an achievement worth celebrating. The journey may not be linear, and there will be challenges, but the potential improvements in mood, focus, behavior, and overall happiness are well worth the commitment.

The journey of introducing a GFCF (gluten-free, casein-free) diet into your child's life is one of dedication, love, and the desire to give them the best opportunity for health and well-being. As a parent or caregiver, the decision to modify your child's diet can feel overwhelming at first, but it can also be incredibly rewarding when you begin to see the positive changes that may follow.

The GFCF diet is an increasingly popular approach for children, particularly those on the autism spectrum or dealing with ADHD, digestive issues, and other developmental challenges. While the diet has gained significant attention in Western countries, it is important to recognize that it can be applied in any culture around the world. Whether you are from a traditionally Arabic, Indian, or Chinese background—or are simply passionate about exploring global cuisines while adhering to the GFCF lifestyle—this book provides the tools you need to adapt traditional flavors and beloved recipes to fit dietary needs without losing their cultural essence.

Arabic cuisine, with its emphasis on fresh vegetables, meats, and rice, naturally offers many dishes that can be adapted to a GFCF diet. Classic staples like hummus, grilled meats, and vegetable stews can be easily made without gluten or dairy. This book offers tips on how to modify traditional Arabic dishes while still honoring the flavors that have been passed down through generations.

Indian cuisine, known for its rich spices and hearty rice and legume-based dishes, also offers a plethora of GFCF-friendly options. While dairy is often used in Indian cooking, substitutions like coconut milk or almond-based yogurt make it possible to enjoy traditional recipes like dal, biryani, and chana masala without compromising on flavor or nutritional value.

For those who appreciate Chinese cuisine, you will find that many dishes are naturally gluten- and dairy-free. With simple modifications like using tamari instead of soy sauce and replacing wheat noodles with rice noodles, it's entirely possible to enjoy the delicious tastes of stir-fries, rice dishes, and steamed meals while maintaining the integrity of a GFCF diet.

This book is designed to help you navigate these cultural traditions and create delicious, nutritious meals that meet the needs of your child while also celebrating the rich culinary history of Arabic, Indian, and Chinese cuisines. As you read through the chapters, you'll find practical advice on how to make these diets work in your own kitchen, dining out, and even while traveling the world.

Embracing the GFCF lifestyle doesn't mean sacrificing the joy and warmth that food can bring. By adapting your cultural favorites to be gluten- and dairy-free, you can continue to share the love of cooking and eating with your family, while supporting their health and well-being in a meaningful way.

I hope this guide serves as an anchor of support, offering clarity, motivation, and hope as you embark on this path. You are not alone in this journey. This book is your companion to help navigate the way, holding your hand through each step toward a healthier, brighter, and more empowered future for your child.

With sincere hope and encouragement,

Tiina Hoddy

CHAPTER 1: Understanding the GFCF Diet and Its Potential Benefits

The decision to make dietary changes for your child is significant, particularly when those changes involve eliminating entire food groups. The GFCF (gluten-free, casein-free) diet is a specialized eating plan that has gained attention for its potential benefits for children, particularly those on the autism spectrum. This chapter will explore what the GFCF diet is, the science behind it, how it can impact your child, and practical steps for getting started

What Is the GFCF Diet?

The GFCF diet involves removing gluten and casein—proteins found in many everyday foods—from a person's diet. Gluten is present in wheat, barley, rye, and foods containing these grains. Casein, on the other hand, is found in dairy products. For children following a GFCF diet, common staples like bread, pasta, milk, and cheese are replaced with gluten- and dairy-free alternatives.

The rise in the popularity of the GFCF diet stems from its perceived benefits for children with autism spectrum disorder (ASD), ADHD, and other developmental delays. While scientific evidence is still evolving, many parents report improvements in behavior, focus, and health, making it an attractive option for those seeking alternative or complementary treatments for their children.

Adopting a GFCF diet can seem daunting at first, but with careful planning, it is possible to replace traditional foods with safe and nutritious alternatives. The next sections will delve deeper into the science behind the GFCF diet, the potential benefits, and the challenges you might encounter as you make the transition.

Historical Context and Origin of the GFCF Diet

The GFCF diet first gained attention in the 1960s and 1970s when researchers began exploring connections between diet and behavior in children with developmental disorders. The idea of modifying diet to improve symptoms became more mainstream in the 1990s when parents and practitioners started sharing anecdotal evidence about how eliminating gluten and casein seemed to improve their children's behavior and overall well-being.

Early studies found that some children with autism exhibited unusual gastrointestinal problems or food sensitivities, which led scientists to explore possible links between diet and symptoms. Researchers hypothesized that the body's inability to properly digest gluten and casein could create abnormal protein breakdown products (called peptides) that might affect brain function. This theory sparked interest in the GFCF diet as a potential intervention.

In the 1990s, families began reporting improvements in their children's mood, social skills, and communication abilities after removing gluten and dairy from their diets. These anecdotal reports helped bring the GFCF diet into the spotlight as a possible treatment for children with autism. While scientific studies have provided mixed results, compelling personal stories and testimonials from families have kept the GFCF diet at the forefront of alternative approaches to supporting children with autism.

The Science Behind the GFCF Diet

As mentioned above the GFCF diet is based on the theory that some children with autism and related disorders may have difficulty digesting gluten and casein. When these proteins are broken down, they produce peptides that, in some children, may act like opiates in the brain. This can potentially interfere with cognitive function, behavior, and overall development.

The "leaky gut" hypothesis suggests that in some children, the intestinal lining is more permeable, allowing these peptides to pass into the bloodstream and affect the brain. This concept is supported by some studies, though it remains a topic of debate. Research in this area continues, as more studies are exploring whether these peptides play a role in the symptoms of autism and how the GFCF diet may affect children's neurological development.

Although not all experts agree on the extent of the impact, some studies have shown that children with autism may have different responses to gluten and casein than neurotypical children. These findings, combined with reports from parents, support the idea that a GFCF diet may be worth exploring if you suspect your child is affected by these proteins. Parents have also reported improvements in behavioral and emotional regulation, suggesting that dietary interventions like the GFCF diet could be an important component of a comprehensive treatment plan for children with autism.

Signs That Your Child Might Benefit from a GFCF Diet
Identifying whether your child might benefit from a GFCF diet involves paying attention to both physical and behavioral signs. Some indicators that could suggest a sensitivity to gluten or casein include:

17

- Chronic Digestive Issues: Frequent bloating, diarrhea, constipation, or stomach pain can often be linked to sensitivities to gluten and casein. Children with autism may have a higher incidence of gastrointestinal issues than neurotypical children.

- Behavioral Changes: Increased irritability, hyperactivity, or meltdowns that seem to occur after eating specific foods. Some children experience behavioral outbursts following the consumption of gluten or dairy products.

- Poor Sleep Quality: Difficulty falling or staying asleep, which may impact daytime behavior and focus. Sleep disturbances are common in children with autism, and dietary interventions may help alleviate these issues.

- Skin Conditions: Recurring rashes or eczema that could be linked to dietary sensitivities. Many children with food sensitivities experience skin reactions.

- Speech and Communication Delays: Some parents have observed improvements in their child's language and communication after removing gluten and casein from their diet.

It's important to note that while these signs can suggest a sensitivity, they do not guarantee that the GFCF diet will work for every child. Consulting with a pediatrician or dietitian who understands dietary interventions can provide guidance on whether this approach might be beneficial. Additionally, ruling out other underlying health conditions is important before starting any new dietary regimen.

Preparing for the Transition to a GFCF Diet

Transitioning to a GFCF diet requires careful planning and preparation. Start by gradually reducing the amount of gluten and dairy in your child's meals while introducing gluten- and dairy-free alternatives. This approach can make the transition smoother and help identify any immediate responses your child may have.

Begin with simple swaps, such as replacing dairy milk with a fortified plant-based alternative (like almond or oat milk) and switching out wheat-based products for gluten-free options like rice or quinoa. The key is to make these changes gradually so that your child's body can adapt and avoid overwhelming them with drastic alterations to their diet all at once.

It is also crucial to educate your child about the changes. Explain the diet in an age-appropriate way so they understand why their meals might look different. For younger children, simple explanations such as, "We're trying new foods to help your tummy feel better and make you feel happier," can be effective. Older children might benefit from more detailed explanations, and involving them in meal planning can help them feel included in the process. This involvement not only gives them a sense of control over their diet but also encourages a positive approach to the transition.

Personal Stories and Testimonials

The GFCF diet's impact is best illustrated by real-life stories. Many parents have reported that within weeks or months of transitioning their children to a GFCF diet, they noticed significant improvements in behavior, focus, and communication. For instance, one mother shared how her son, who previously struggled with meltdowns and limited verbal communication, became calmer and began using more words to express himself after eliminating gluten and dairy. His teachers even noted improvements in his ability to focus in class.

These stories are supported by an increasing number of families who have seen positive changes. While the experiences vary from child to child, the common thread is the notable shift in behavior, mood, or physical well-being that comes with dietary adjustments. The diet's potential benefits, from reducing digestive discomfort to improving social skills, have encouraged many families to give the GFCF approach a try.

However, it is important to note that not every child experiences drastic changes. While many families report positive results, others may see only subtle improvements or no noticeable change at all. This variability highlights the importance of approaching the GFCF diet as one part of a broader approach to health and wellness, recognizing that what works for one child may not work for another

Initial Expectations and Adjustments

It's important to set realistic expectations when beginning the GFCF diet. Some children may show improvements within weeks, while for others, it may take months. During the initial phase, parents may notice withdrawal-like symptoms as the body adjusts to the absence of gluten and casein. These symptoms could include irritability, restlessness, or changes in appetite.

For example, some children may experience a temporary increase in behavioral issues as the body detoxes from gluten and dairy. This phase, though challenging, is often temporary. Keep a food and behavior journal to document what your child eats and any changes you observe. This will help you track patterns, identify improvements, and make necessary adjustments. If progress seems slow, don't be discouraged; every child's body responds differently, and persistence is key.

One common challenge in the beginning is finding the right GFCF substitutes. Initially, you may need to try different brands of gluten- and dairy-free products to see what your child enjoys. While some alternatives may be difficult for them to accept at first, others may quickly become new favorites. Patience and experimentation are key to finding a balanced approach that works for your child.

Common Challenges and Solutions

Starting a GFCF diet can come with challenges, such as finding suitable replacements for favorite foods and managing mealtime resistance. Begin by exploring the growing variety of gluten- and dairy-free products available in stores and online. Experiment with different brands and recipes to find what your child enjoys.

Involving your child in meal preparation can make them more receptive to dietary changes. Let them help pick out new foods at the grocery store or assist in simple kitchen tasks. This engagement can make the process feel more exciting and less restrictive. For example, involving your child in making gluten-free pizza with their favorite toppings can make the meal feel familiar and fun.

Another common challenge is managing social situations, such as parties and school events. Pack GFCF-friendly snacks and inform teachers and caregivers about your child's dietary needs to ensure they're supported outside the home. Being proactive and communicating dietary restrictions to schools or event hosts can help prevent any misunderstandings and ensure that your child is included in all social activities.

Preparing Your Kitchen and Pantry

Stocking your kitchen with GFCF staples is an essential part of making the transition smoother. Replace traditional breads, pastas, and cereals with gluten-free versions. For dairy substitutes, explore plant-based milks like almond, coconut, or oat milk, and try dairy-free cheeses and yogurts. Keep a range of fresh fruits, vegetables, lean proteins, and gluten-free grains like rice and quinoa on hand.

Label foods in your pantry to avoid cross-contamination, especially if only one member of the family is following the diet. Using separate utensils, cookware, and toasters can help maintain a safe environment for your child. To keep things organized, store gluten-free products on dedicated shelves, separate from regular pantry items, and maintain clear labeling of food items.

The Support System: Building a Community

Transitioning to a GFCF diet is easier when you have a support system. Connect with other parents who have implemented the diet for their children, whether through local groups, online forums, or social media. Sharing recipes, success stories, and challenges can provide valuable insight and encouragement. Engaging with a community helps you feel less isolated and more empowered to make informed decisions.

Participating in these groups allows you to exchange tips on meal planning, find recommendations for GFCF-friendly products, and gain emotional support from others who are on the same journey. For example, some online forums offer specific resources for families with children on the autism spectrum who follow a GFCF diet, providing a wealth of shared experiences and expertise

Moving Forward with Confidence

Embarking on the GFCF journey is an act of dedication to your child's health and well-being. While the transition may seem daunting at first, the potential benefits make it a worthwhile endeavor. Equip yourself with the knowledge, resources, and support you need, and remember that progress takes time. Whether you see significant changes or more subtle improvements, your commitment to trying new approaches can make a meaningful difference in your child's life.

In the next chapter, we will explore how to build balanced, nutrient-rich meals that support overall health while adhering to a GFCF diet. By understanding how to create well-rounded meals, you can ensure your child receives all the essential nutrients they need to thrive on this specialized diet.

CHAPTER 2: Creating Balanced Meals in a GFCF Diet

Transitioning to a GFCF diet for your child is more than just eliminating gluten and dairy; it's about ensuring that the meals they eat are balanced and nutritious. Achieving a proper nutritional balance helps support growth, cognitive development, and overall health, especially for children who may already have specific dietary needs. This chapter will explore the essential components of balanced meals within this diet, practical tips for meal planning, and examples of nutrient-rich meals.

The Importance of Balanced Nutrition in a GFCF Diet

Balanced nutrition is key for any child, but it becomes even more critical when certain food groups are eliminated. Gluten and dairy are often significant sources of vitamins and minerals, such as calcium and B vitamins. When these food groups are removed, it's essential to replace them with alternatives that provide equivalent nutritional value. Balanced meals help support energy levels, mood stability, and cognitive function, laying the foundation for a healthy, active life.

A balanced meal in a GFCF diet should include:

- Proteins for growth and muscle development.

- Healthy fats for brain health and hormone production.

- Complex carbohydrates for sustained energy.

- Vitamins and minerals to support overall well-being.

Understanding these components and incorporating them into your child's diet can make meal planning easier and more effective.

Nutrient-Rich GFCF Food Groups
When planning GFCF meals, focus on nutrient-dense foods that provide a variety of essential vitamins and minerals. Here are some key food groups and examples of options that fit within a GFCF diet:

Proteins
Protein is crucial for growth, immune function, and muscle repair. In a GFCF diet, protein sources should be diverse to ensure adequate intake. Consider:

- Lean Meats: Chicken, turkey, and lean cuts of beef or pork.

- Fish: Salmon, mackerel, and sardines, which also provide omega-3 fatty acids.

- Eggs: A versatile protein source that can be included in various meals.

- Legumes: Beans, lentils, and chickpeas are plant-based protein sources that are also rich in fiber.

- Nuts and Seeds: Almonds, sunflower seeds, and chia seeds provide both protein and healthy fats.

Healthy Fats

Fats play an important role in brain health, energy, and the absorption of fat-soluble vitamins (A, D, E, and K). GFCF-friendly healthy fats include:

- Avocado: A great source of monounsaturated fats.

- Olive Oil: Ideal for dressings and light cooking.

- Coconut Oil: A versatile cooking oil with a unique flavor profile.

- Nut Butters: Almond butter and sunflower seed butter can be spread on gluten-free bread or used in recipes.

- Fatty Fish: Salmon and mackerel provide both protein and healthy omega-3 Naturally gluten-free options.

Complex Carbohydrates

Complex carbohydrates provide sustained energy and are rich in fiber, which aids digestion. Options that are naturally gluten-free include:

Whole Grains Vegetables and Fruits

- Brown rice, quinoa, millet, and gluten-free oats.

- Starchy Vegetables: Sweet potatoes, butternut squash, and plantains.

- Legumes: Chickpeas and lentils double as protein and complex carbs.

- Fruits: Bananas, apples, and berries offer natural sweetness and essential vitamins.

These are essential for providing a wide range of vitamins, minerals, and antioxidants. Aim for a colorful variety to maximize nutrient intake:

- Leafy Greens: Spinach, kale, and Swiss chard are rich in iron and vitamin K.

- Cruciferous Vegetables: Broccoli, cauliflower, and Brussels sprouts offer fiber and phytonutrients.

- Brightly Colored Vegetables: Carrots, bell peppers, and tomatoes add vitamin A and vitamin C.

- Fruits: Berries, citrus fruits, and apples are excellent sources of vitamins and fiber.

Meal Composition and Portion Sizes

Structuring meals in a balanced way ensures your child receives a variety of nutrients. A simple guideline for portioning meals is to divide the plate into three main sections:

- Half the plate should be filled with vegetables and fruits.

- A quarter of the plate should include lean proteins.

- The remaining quarter should contain complex carbohydrates or grains.

- A serving of healthy fats can be incorporated as a dressing, cooking oil, or added ingredient.

Addressing Potential Nutritional Gaps

While the GFCF diet can be nutritious, there are a few nutrients that may require special attention to prevent deficiencies:

Calcium and Vitamin D

Without dairy, calcium and vitamin D intake might be lower. To address this:

- Include calcium-fortified dairy-free milk (e.g., almond, oat, or soy milk).

- Add leafy greens like kale and bok choy to meals.

- Ensure exposure to sunlight for natural vitamin D or consider a vitamin D supplement, after consulting with a healthcare provider.

B Vitamins

Whole grains often provide B vitamins, so be sure to incorporate fortified gluten-free cereals and a variety of fruits and vegetables. Eggs, meat, and legumes are also good sources of B vitamins.

Iron and Zinc

Iron is found in both plant and animal sources, but heme iron (from animal sources) is more readily absorbed. Include lean meats, poultry, and fortified gluten-free cereals to boost iron intake. For plant-based options, pair iron-rich foods like lentils with vitamin C sources to enhance absorption.

Practical Tips for Meal Planning and Preparation

Planning balanced GFCF meals can seem daunting at first, but it becomes manageable with a few strategies:

- Batch Cooking: Prepare larger portions of GFCF staples like quinoa, rice, or grilled chicken to save time during the week.

- Grocery Shopping: Make a shopping list of GFCF essentials, including fresh produce, gluten-free grains, and protein sources. This can streamline your grocery trips and ensure you always have what you need.

- Weekly Menus: Plan meals for the week in advance to avoid last-minute scrambling. Rotate different proteins and vegetables to keep meals varied and nutritionally complete.

Building a GFCF Pantry

Stocking your pantry with GFCF essentials will make meal preparation easier. Here are items to consider:

- Gluten-Free Flours: Almond flour, coconut flour, and rice flour for baking and cooking.

- Gluten-Free Grains: Brown rice, quinoa, millet, and gluten-free pasta.

- Plant-Based Milk: Almond milk, coconut milk, and oat milk, preferably fortified.

- Dairy-Free Cheese: Nutritional yeast or dairy-free cheese alternatives for flavor and texture.

- Healthy Oils: Olive oil, coconut oil, and avocado oil for cooking and dressings.

- Nuts and Seeds: Almonds, chia seeds, flaxseeds, and sunflower seeds for snacks and recipes.

- Legumes: Canned or dried beans, lentils, and chickpeas for protein and fiber.

Balancing Convenience and Nutrition

Busy days call for quick solutions that don't compromise on nutrition. Keep healthy, pre-packaged GFCF snacks on hand, such as gluten-free protein bars, fruit leathers, or dairy-free yogurts. On days when time is tight, a simple plate of scrambled eggs with spinach or a bowl of rice and beans can provide balanced nutrition without much effort.

Final Thoughts

Ensuring your child's meals are balanced and nutritious within a GFCF diet requires thought, but it is achievable with the right strategies. By incorporating a variety of proteins, healthy fats, complex carbohydrates, and nutrient-rich vegetables and fruits, you can create meals that support your child's health and well-being. Planning, stocking a well-prepared pantry, and having go-to meal ideas can make maintaining a balanced diet easier and more enjoyable for the whole family.

In the next chapter, we will dive into practical recipes and tips for preparing GFCF meals that your child will love, making mealtimes smoother and more enjoyable for everyone involved.

CHAPTER 3: Navigating the Transition to a GFCF Diet

Transitioning to a GFCF diet can feel significant for any family. Knowing how to make this transition smoothly is essential to ensure your child receives balanced nutrition and feels supported throughout the process. In this chapter, we'll cover practical strategies to make this shift easier, common pitfalls to avoid, tips for reading food labels, and how to handle social situations and dining out. With these strategies, you can create a seamless experience that benefits your child's health and overall well-being.

Starting a GFCF diet can be daunting, and it's easy to make a few common mistakes in the beginning. One of the most frequent mistakes is not reading ingredient labels carefully. It's common to assume that a product labeled as "gluten-free" is also free of casein, or vice versa, but gluten and dairy can be hidden in unexpected places. Ingredients like malt (which contains gluten), whey (a dairy byproduct), and modified food starch (potentially derived from wheat) can be overlooked.

Another common issue is relying too heavily on packaged gluten-free foods. These products can be convenient but are often highly processed and lacking in nutrients. Overreliance on them can result in a diet that is low in fiber and high in sugars or unhealthy fats. Strive to include whole, unprocessed foods as much as possible to provide the best nutrition.

Cross-contamination is another significant concern. In kitchens where gluten-containing and gluten-free foods are prepared together, it's easy for cross-contact to occur. This can happen if the same cutting boards, toasters, or utensils are used for both types of food, which can introduce gluten into an otherwise gluten-free meal.

Reading food labels effectively is crucial for maintaining a strict GFCF diet. Ingredients lists can be confusing, with hidden sources of gluten and casein appearing under different names. For gluten, watch for hidden sources such as malt, which is found in malt vinegar and syrup, barley in cereals, and modified food starch, which could be wheat-derived unless specified as gluten-free. For casein, hidden sources include whey, curds used in cheeses, caseinate found in processed foods, and products labeled as "lactose-free," which may still contain casein. Always check for allergen warnings like "Contains: Wheat" or "Contains: Milk," and be cautious with "vegan" labels, which may be dairy-free but not necessarily gluten-free.

Cross-contamination can make a GFCF diet ineffective and lead to unintended reactions. To prevent this, use separate utensils and cookware designated for gluten-free cooking and label them to avoid confusion. Clean kitchen surfaces thoroughly before preparing GFCF meals, especially if they're also used for gluten or dairy-containing foods. Store GFCF foods in dedicated containers or sections of your pantry and refrigerator to minimize the risk of contamination.

Dining out while maintaining a GFCF diet can be challenging, but with some planning, it's manageable. Research restaurants that cater to gluten-free and dairy-free diets and check their menus online. When at a restaurant, communicate clearly with the server about dietary restrictions using specific phrases like, "We need a meal that is gluten-free and dairy-free with no cross-contamination." Don't hesitate to ask how food is prepared and if separate utensils and surfaces are used. To be safe, bring along GFCF-friendly snacks such as gluten-free crackers, fruit, or dairy-free yogurt in case the menu options are limited.

Stocking your kitchen with GFCF essentials makes meal preparation easier and more efficient. Include staple ingredients like gluten-free flour (almond, coconut, rice flour), dairy-free milk (almond, coconut, oat, soy milk), gluten-free grains (quinoa, brown rice, oats), legumes, and nut butters. As discussed before, tools for preventing cross-contamination, can help maintain a safe cooking environment.

Transitioning your child to a GFCF diet is easier when the whole family is involved. Inclusive meal planning that everyone can enjoy minimizes feelings of exclusion and encourages family support. Educate and engage siblings so they understand the diet's importance and how they can help. Make it a team effort by involving siblings in meal prep or teaching them to look for gluten-free and dairy-free labels. Turn meal preparation into an enjoyable activity by experimenting with new GFCF recipes together. Let your child choose a dish to try or create themed meal nights like "Taco Tuesday" with gluten-free tortillas and dairy-free toppings.

GFCF foods can sometimes be more expensive, but there are ways to manage the cost. Buying in bulk helps save money on staples like gluten-free flours, rice, and legumes. Using seasonal produce is another way to get better pricing and nutritional value. Homemade alternatives, like baking your own GFCF bread or snacks, can also reduce costs and give you control over the ingredients. Visiting farmers' markets can provide fresh produce at potentially lower prices.

Balancing a busy schedule while preparing GFCF meals is challenging but achievable with the right strategies. Batch cooking larger quantities of GFCF meals and freezing portions can save time during the week. Slow cookers and Instant Pots are perfect for hands-off meal preparation, allowing you to make GFCF soups, stews, and casseroles with minimal effort. Prepping ingredients in stages, like chopping vegetables or marinating proteins ahead of time, makes daily cooking faster and easier.

Adapting family favorite recipes to be GFCF-friendly helps maintain a sense of normalcy at mealtimes. Replace all-purpose flour with gluten-free flour blends that often include rice flour, tapioca starch, and xanthan gum for better texture. Swap dairy milk for almond or coconut milk and use dairy-free cheese or nutritional yeast for a cheesy flavor. For soups and sauces, cornstarch, arrowroot powder, or potato starch can be used as thickening agents instead of flour.

Finding support systems and resources can make transitioning to a GFCF diet more manageable. Join online communities where parents share recipes, tips, and encouragement, and follow GFCF food blogs for recipe inspiration and product reviews. Connecting with local support groups or attending workshops can offer additional guidance and the chance to network with parents facing similar challenges.

CHAPTER 4: Building Balanced GFCF Meal Plans

Creating balanced, nutritious meal plans is essential when following a GFCF diet. The goal is to ensure that your child receives a wide range of nutrients to support their physical health, cognitive function, and emotional well-being. This chapter will cover how to build a meal plan that includes a variety of proteins, healthy fats, complex carbohydrates, and fresh produce, while also addressing potential nutritional gaps. You'll find practical meal-planning strategies, tips for rotating meals to avoid monotony, and ideas for incorporating diverse flavors and textures.

Transitioning to a GFCF diet can feel restrictive at first, but with a thoughtful approach, it's possible to create meal plans that are both nutritious and enjoyable. Balanced meal planning starts with understanding the essential components of a healthy diet. Each meal should include a combination of proteins, healthy fats, and carbohydrates, as well as vitamins and minerals from vegetables and fruits. This approach ensures sustained energy, supports growth, and promotes overall well-being.

Essential Components of a Balanced GFCF Meal

Proteins are the building blocks of the body, vital for growth, muscle repair, and immune function. In a GFCF diet, protein sources should be varied to maintain interest and nutritional diversity. Options include lean meats such as chicken, turkey, and beef, as well as fish like salmon and mackerel, which are rich in omega-3 fatty acids. Eggs, legumes such as beans and lentils, and plant-based proteins like tofu are also great additions. Nuts and seeds, including almonds, sunflower seeds, and pumpkin seeds, can be included as snacks or incorporated into meals.

Healthy fats are essential for brain development, hormone production, and the absorption of fat-soluble vitamins (A, D, E, and K). Good sources of healthy fats for a GFCF diet include avocados, olive oil, and coconut oil. Fatty fish such as salmon provides a dual benefit of protein and omega-3 fatty acids. Nut butters, like almond and sunflower seed butter, can be spread on gluten-free bread or added to smoothies for a nutritional boost.

Complex carbohydrates are an important energy source, providing the fuel needed for daily activities. Gluten-free grains such as quinoa, brown rice, and millet are excellent options that also contribute fiber to the diet. Starchy vegetables like sweet potatoes, butternut squash, and plantains are nutrient-dense sources of complex carbs. Legumes, which also double as a protein source, provide sustained energy and essential vitamins.

Vegetables and fruits are packed with vitamins, minerals, and antioxidants. Aiming for a colorful variety ensures that your child receives a broad spectrum of nutrients. Leafy greens such as spinach and kale are rich in iron and vitamin K, while brightly colored vegetables like carrots and bell peppers provide vitamins A and C. Fruits like berries, apples, and citrus offer vitamins, fiber, and natural sweetness.

Creating a weekly meal plan can save time and reduce stress. Start by mapping out meals for breakfast, lunch, dinner, and snacks. Rotate proteins, vegetables, and grains throughout the week to ensure nutritional diversity and prevent boredom. For example, include grilled chicken with brown rice and steamed broccoli one day, and switch to baked salmon with quinoa and sautéed spinach the next.

Focus on Whole Foods

While gluten-free packaged foods can be convenient, they often lack the nutrients provided by whole foods. Prioritize meals that include fresh produce, lean proteins, and natural fats. Incorporating whole foods helps maintain energy levels and supports overall health.

Batch Cooking and Meal Prep

Prepping meals in advance can make following a GFCF diet more manageable, especially for busy families. Prepare larger batches of staple foods like quinoa, brown rice, or grilled chicken, and store them in the refrigerator or freezer. This allows you to mix and match components throughout the week to create balanced meals without daily cooking. Soups and stews made with GFCF ingredients can also be made in bulk and reheated as needed.

Incorporate Snacks

Healthy snacks can help maintain energy levels between meals and prevent hunger. Simple snack ideas include sliced apples with almond butter, carrot sticks with hummus, or homemade trail mix with dried fruit and pumpkin seeds. These snacks are easy to prepare and provide a blend of proteins, fats, and carbohydrates.

Simple, Balanced GFCF Meal Ideas

Here are examples of balanced GFCF meals that you can easily prepare:

Breakfast

- Smoothie Bowl: Blend frozen bananas, spinach, and dairy-free milk. Top with chia seeds, berries, and a sprinkle of gluten-free granola.

- Egg Muffins: Whisk eggs with chopped spinach, dairy-free cheese, and diced tomatoes. Bake in a muffin tin for an easy grab-and-go breakfast.

- Overnight Oats: Use gluten-free oats soaked in coconut milk, topped with fresh fruit and sunflower seeds.

Lunch

- Quinoa Salad: Combine cooked quinoa with cherry tomatoes, cucumber, chickpeas, and a drizzle of olive oil and lemon juice.

- Turkey Lettuce Wraps: Fill large lettuce leaves with sliced turkey, avocado, shredded carrots, and hummus.

Dinner

- Salmon and Sweet Potatoes: Roast salmon with olive oil and herbs, paired with baked sweet potatoes and steamed broccoli.

- Grilled Chicken and Sweet Potato: Serve with a side of steamed green beans.

- Salmon with Brown Rice: Pair with roasted Brussels sprouts and a drizzle of lemon juice.

- Stir-Fry: Sauté chicken, bell peppers, broccoli, and snap peas in coconut oil with gluten-free tamari or coconut aminos. Serve over rice.

Snacks

- Fruit and Nut Mix: A mix of almonds, dried cranberries, and sunflower seeds.

- Veggies with Hummus: Carrot sticks, cucumber slices, and celery served with dairy-free hummus.

Meal Rotation and Variety

To prevent mealtime monotony, rotate different proteins, vegetables, and grains throughout the week. Introduce new foods regularly to expand your child's palate and nutrition profile. Trying new recipes can be a fun family activity and encourages children to be more open to different tastes and textures.

Tips for Incorporating Diverse Flavors and Textures

Children can be more willing to try new foods when meals offer a variety of flavors and textures. Incorporate spices and herbs such as basil, cilantro, and cinnamon to add depth to meals without gluten or dairy. Experiment with different cooking methods, such as roasting vegetables for a caramelized flavor or sautéing greens for a tender texture.

Practical Meal Planning Tips

Keep meals simple and balanced by focusing on one protein source, one carbohydrate, and a selection of vegetables. For instance, a dinner of grilled chicken, brown rice, and roasted carrots provides a mix of protein, fiber, vitamins, and minerals. Aim to prep ingredients that can be used in multiple meals to cut down on cooking time. For example, cook extra quinoa to use as a base for both lunch salads and dinner side dishes.

Final Thoughts

Balanced meal planning on a GFCF diet ensures that your child receives the nutrition they need while enjoying varied and delicious meals. By focusing on diverse food groups, planning ahead, and keeping meals interesting, you can create an environment where healthy eating becomes a sustainable and enjoyable part of life. The effort you invest in meal planning not only supports your child's health but also fosters a positive relationship with food. In the next chapter, we'll look at strategies to make GFCF eating more enjoyable for your child and practical ways to deal with picky eating

CHAPTER 5: Making GFCF Eating Enjoyable for Your Child

Adopting a GFCF (gluten-free, casein-free) diet can be a significant change for children, especially those who may already have strong food preferences or sensory sensitivities. Ensuring that the transition is positive and enjoyable is essential to creating a sustainable eating plan. This chapter will cover strategies for making GFCF meals appealing to your child, tips for overcoming resistance, and ways to introduce variety while maintaining the diet.

Children, especially those on the autism spectrum, often thrive on routine. Shifting to a GFCF diet may disrupt their sense of comfort, especially if favorite foods are suddenly off-limits. It's important to approach this transition with patience and creativity to encourage a positive association with the new way of eating.

Children may resist new foods due to unfamiliar textures, tastes, or colors. It's essential to understand that this resistance is normal and can be managed with consistent, supportive strategies. Making GFCF meals fun and engaging can turn what might initially be met with hesitation into an exciting culinary adventure.

Making GFCF Meals More Appealing

1. Get Creative with Presentation

Presentation plays an important role in how children perceive their food. Meals that are visually appealing are more likely to be received with enthusiasm. Use cookie cutters to shape sandwiches or pancakes into fun characters or animals. Arrange fruits and vegetables into colorful patterns or smiley faces on the plate.

2. Incorporate Familiar Flavors

When introducing new GFCF foods, pair them with familiar flavors that your child already enjoys. For instance, if your child loves peanut butter, try serving it with gluten-free crackers or sliced apples. Using familiar seasonings like cinnamon, garlic, or mild herbs can help bridge the gap between old favorites and new options.

3. Make Mealtimes Interactive

Involving your child in meal preparation can make them more interested in trying what they've helped create. Let them stir, mix, or choose ingredients. This hands-on experience builds curiosity and encourages them to taste the final dish.

4. Introduce Changes Gradually

If your child is particularly sensitive to changes, introduce new GFCF foods one at a time and incorporate them into familiar meals. For example, serve gluten-free pasta with a sauce they already love. Gradual changes can help build acceptance and reduce resistance.

Tips for Overcoming Resistance

Overcoming initial resistance requires a combination of patience and consistency. Here are some tips to help:
- Start Small: Begin with small portions of new foods and gradually increase the amount as your child becomes accustomed to the taste and texture.

- Positive Reinforcement: Praise your child for trying new foods, even if they only take a small bite. Positive reinforcement helps them associate new experiences with success.

- Model Behavior: Eat the same GFCF meals as your child to show them that the whole family can enjoy the diet. Children often mimic the behavior of their parents and siblings.

- Create a Calm Eating Environment: Reducing distractions during mealtimes can help children focus on their food and feel more relaxed about trying new dishes.

Introducing Variety into GFCF Meals

A GFCF diet can sometimes feel limiting, especially at first. However, there are many ways to keep meals interesting and varied:

Different cultures offer a range of naturally gluten-free and dairy-free foods. For instance, Mexican cuisine features corn tortillas and rice dishes, while many Thai recipes include coconut milk instead of dairy. Exploring world cuisines can introduce new flavors and textures that excite your child's palate. Changing how you prepare familiar ingredients can make a big difference. For example, roasting vegetables can bring out their natural sweetness, while steaming or sautéing can create softer, more appealing textures. Try baking sweet potatoes as fries or blending them into a creamy dairy-free soup. Turn mealtime into a special event by incorporating themes, such as "Rainbow Day" where each part of the meal features a different color of the rainbow, or "Taco Night" with gluten-free taco shells and a variety of fillings. Themed meals can make the dining experience feel unique and exciting.

Dealing with Sensory Sensitivities

Many children, particularly those on the autism spectrum, may have sensory sensitivities that affect their willingness to try new foods. These sensitivities can involve taste, texture, temperature, or even the smell of certain foods. Observe your child's reactions to different textures and flavors. Some children prefer crunchy foods, while others might enjoy soft or smooth textures. Knowing these preferences can guide your meal planning and help make new foods more appealing. Giving your child choices empowers them and makes them feel involved in the process. Present a few GFCF options and let them pick which one they'd like to try. This can reduce resistance and encourage them to engage with their meals.

If your child struggles with certain textures, try modifying the way foods are prepared. Pureeing vegetables into soups or sauces, cutting fruits into smaller pieces, or serving foods at different temperatures (warm, room temperature, or cold) can help make them more palatable.

Making mealtimes enjoyable is key to long-term success with a GFCF diet. Reducing pressure and maintaining a relaxed atmosphere can help your child associate food with positive experiences. If your child refuses a new food, avoid forcing them to eat it. Instead, reintroduce it at a later date and in a different way. Consistency without pressure helps children become more open to trying new foods over time.

When the whole family participates in eating GFCF meals, your child is less likely to feel singled out. Family meals create a supportive environment and show that everyone is sharing in the experience.

Serving food on colorful plates or with fun-shaped utensils can make mealtime more inviting. Little touches like using animal-shaped forks or plates with characters can create excitement around eating.

Final Thoughts

Transitioning to a GFCF diet doesn't have to mean losing out on enjoyable meals. With a little creativity and patience, mealtimes can become a time of discovery and joy for your child. By making small changes, being consistent, and involving your child in the process, you can help them develop a positive relationship with their food. The goal is not just adherence to the diet but creating a healthy, balanced eating routine that your child looks forward to. In the next chapter, we will explore practical ways to keep your GFCF diet balanced and nutritious as your child's tastes and dietary needs evolve

CHAPTER 6: Keeping a GFCF Diet Balanced and Nutritious

Maintaining a balanced and nutritious GFCF (gluten-free, casein-free) diet is essential to support the overall health, growth, and development of your child. This chapter explores how to ensure that meals provide the necessary macronutrients, fiber, vitamins, and minerals while staying within the GFCF guidelines. By implementing these strategies, you can help your child thrive on a GFCF diet without compromising nutritional quality.

Understanding Macronutrient Balance

Macronutrients—proteins, carbohydrates, and fats—are the foundation of a balanced diet. Each plays a vital role in your child's health:

Proteins

Proteins are essential for growth, muscle repair, and immune function. In a GFCF diet, you can include lean meats such as chicken and turkey, fish rich in omega-3s like salmon, eggs, legumes, tofu, and dairy-free protein powders. Ensuring a variety of protein sources helps maintain interest and provides a wide range of amino acids.

Carbohydrates

Carbohydrates provide the energy needed for daily activities. Opt for complex carbohydrates that are rich in fiber and nutrients, such as gluten-free whole grains (brown rice, quinoa, millet), starchy vegetables (sweet potatoes, squash), and legumes. These options supply energy steadily throughout the day, avoiding the quick spikes and crashes often associated with simple carbohydrates.

Fats

Fats are necessary for brain health, hormone production, and the absorption of fat-soluble vitamins (A, D, E, and K). Incorporate healthy fats such as avocados, olive oil, coconut oil, and fatty fish. Nut butters, such as almond and sunflower seed butter, can be added to meals or snacks for an extra nutritional boost.

Fiber

Ensuring Adequate Fiber Intake

Fiber is crucial for digestive health, yet gluten-free products can sometimes lack sufficient fiber. To ensure your child receives adequate fiber, focus on including:

- Fruits and Vegetables: Apples, berries, pears, carrots, broccoli, and spinach are high in fiber and rich in vitamins.

- Legumes: Lentils, chickpeas, and black beans provide both protein and fiber.

- Gluten-Free Whole Grains: Quinoa, brown rice, and gluten-free oats are excellent sources of fiber.

These foods not only support healthy digestion but also help regulate blood sugar levels and keep your child feeling full longer.

Maintaining a Healthy Gut

A balanced gut microbiome is essential for digestion and overall health. This is particularly important for children on the autism spectrum, who may experience more digestive issues. A GFCF diet can support gut health when supplemented with:

- Probiotic-Rich Foods: Options such as dairy-free yogurt with active cultures, fermented vegetables (sauerkraut or kimchi), and dairy-free kefir can help maintain a healthy gut flora.

- Prebiotic Foods: Garlic, onions, bananas, and asparagus can nourish beneficial gut bacteria and improve digestion.

Ensuring a balance of probiotics and prebiotics in your child's diet helps enhance nutrient absorption and supports their immune system.

Navigating Nutritional Gaps

While a GFCF diet can be nutritious, certain nutrients may be less abundant, especially if dairy and fortified grains were significant sources. Here's how to address potential nutritional gaps:

Calcium and Vitamin D

Without dairy, calcium intake needs to be supplemented through fortified plant-based milks like almond or oat milk, leafy greens such as kale and bok choy, and fish like canned salmon with bones. Vitamin D is crucial for calcium absorption and can be more challenging to obtain through diet alone. Ensure your child has regular sunlight exposure, and consider vitamin D supplements if needed, after consulting with a healthcare provider.

B Vitamins

B vitamins are vital for energy production and brain health. Include eggs, poultry, gluten-free fortified cereals, and a range of vegetables to maintain adequate intake. Beans and lentils are also rich in B vitamins and fiber, making them valuable additions to the diet.

Iron and Zinc

Iron supports oxygen transport in the blood, while zinc plays a role in immune health. Lean meats, poultry, and seafood are good sources of both nutrients. For plant-based options, include iron-rich foods like spinach and lentils, and pair them with vitamin C sources like bell peppers or strawberries to enhance iron absorption.

The Importance of Hydration

Proper hydration is often overlooked but is essential for a balanced diet. Water aids in digestion helps maintain energy levels, and supports cognitive function. Encourage your child to drink water throughout the day, and incorporate hydrating snacks such as watermelon, cucumbers, and oranges. Herbal teas and infused water with fruit can make hydration more appealing to children who are reluctant to drink plain water.

Mindful Eating Practices

Teaching children to practice mindful eating can help them recognize hunger cues, appreciate their meals, and develop healthy eating habits. Mindful eating involves:

- Encouraging Slower Eating: Teach your child to take smaller bites and chew thoroughly. This helps them recognize when they are full and promotes better digestion.

- Creating a Calm Eating Environment: A distraction-free space allows children to focus on their food and enjoy mealtime.

- Engaging in Conversations: Talking about flavors and textures can make mealtimes more interactive and help children develop a greater appreciation for their food.

Seasonal Eating for Nutritional Variety

Eating seasonally not only supports local farmers but also ensures a variety of nutrients throughout the year. Seasonal produce is often fresher and more nutrient-dense. For example, summer offers berries, zucchini, and bell peppers, while winter provides hearty vegetables like sweet potatoes and Brussels sprouts. Adjusting meal plans to include seasonal ingredients helps keep meals diverse and exciting.

Balancing Plant-Based and Animal-Based Foods

Families looking to incorporate more plant-based meals into their GFCF diet can do so while maintaining nutritional balance. Plant-based proteins such as lentils, quinoa, and chickpeas can be rotated with animal-based proteins like chicken and fish. This balance supports a varied intake of essential amino acids and nutrients.

Fun Ways to Incorporate Nutrient-Dense Foods
Introducing nutrient-dense foods in creative ways can help make meals more appealing to children. Here are some ideas:

- Smoothies: Blend leafy greens like spinach or kale with bananas, berries, and dairy-free milk for a tasty and nutrient-packed drink.

- Baked Goods: Add ground flaxseed or chia seeds to GFCF muffins or pancakes for an omega-3 and fiber boost.

- Hidden Vegetables: Incorporate pureed vegetables into sauces or soups to enhance nutrient intake without altering the flavor significantly.

Ensuring Nutritional Adequacy in Packed Lunches
Preparing balanced GFCF-packed lunches for school or outings can help maintain consistency and nutrition. Ideas for packed lunches include:

- Quinoa Salad: Mix quinoa with chickpeas, cherry tomatoes, and cucumber for a refreshing and filling meal.

- Rice Cakes with Almond Butter: Top with banana slices for a sweet and satisfying snack.

- Turkey Roll-Ups: Wrap slices of turkey around cucumber sticks or avocado slices for an easy, protein-rich option.

Final Thoughts

Keeping a GFCF diet balanced and nutritious involves understanding how to meet your child's nutritional needs through a variety of foods. By ensuring a balance of macronutrients, addressing potential nutritional gaps, promoting mindful eating, and incorporating diverse and fun foods, you can support your child's health and well-being. The effort you put into planning and maintaining a balanced diet helps create a positive eating experience and contributes to your child's growth and development. In the next chapter, we will explore strategies for keeping the GFCF diet sustainable and adaptable as your child's needs evolve.

CHAPTER 7: Sustaining and Adapting the GFCF Diet

Maintaining a GFCF (gluten-free, casein-free) diet over the long term requires planning, adaptability, and a proactive approach to ensure it continues to meet your child's nutritional and lifestyle needs. As children grow and their dietary preferences and nutritional requirements evolve, parents need strategies to sustain the GFCF diet without it feeling restrictive or monotonous. This chapter will explore how to keep the diet sustainable, adapt it over different life stages, and make it flexible enough for special situations and changing preferences.

Sustaining the GFCF Diet Over Time

One of the keys to sustaining a GFCF diet is to approach it as a long-term lifestyle rather than a temporary change. To prevent meal fatigue, it's important to regularly introduce new recipes and ingredients. Keep meals interesting by experimenting with different cuisines and flavors that are naturally gluten- and casein-free, such as Mediterranean, Thai, or Mexican dishes. Incorporating new herbs, spices, and cooking methods like grilling, roasting, or steaming can also help maintain variety.

Involving the whole family in meal planning not only eases the workload but also reinforces that the GFCF diet is an inclusive part of family life. Let your child have input by choosing ingredients or themes for the week's meals. This makes them feel involved and more likely to be enthusiastic about trying the dishes.

Adapting the Diet for Different Life Stages

As children grow, their nutritional needs change. The GFCF diet must adapt to meet these requirements and match evolving tastes. For younger children, focus on meals that are visually appealing and easy to eat, with softer textures and familiar flavors. As children move into adolescence, their caloric and protein needs may increase due to growth spurts and higher activity levels. Introduce more protein-rich foods like eggs, lean meats, legumes, and dairy-free protein shakes to support these changes.

Teenagers may seek more independence in their food choices. This is a great time to teach them how to make their own GFCF meals and snacks. Help them understand how to read food labels, check for hidden sources of gluten and casein, and prepare balanced meals that fit their taste preferences. Encouraging them to take an active role in meal prep builds confidence and makes the diet more sustainable as they mature.

Making the Diet Flexible

Maintaining flexibility in a GFCF diet can prevent burnout and promote long-term success. Plan for occasional treats and special dishes to make the diet feel less restrictive. This can include making GFCF-friendly versions of favorite comfort foods, such as dairy-free macaroni and cheese or gluten-free pizza. Special occasions, holidays, and celebrations can be enjoyable and inclusive when you prepare or bring GFCF-friendly versions of party foods, such as cupcakes, cookies, and finger foods.

When dining out or traveling, flexibility is key. Research restaurants ahead of time that offer gluten-free and dairy-free options, and don't hesitate to call and ask questions about their ability to accommodate dietary restrictions. If necessary, pack snacks or small meals to ensure your child always has a safe option available.

Building a GFCF Pantry for the Long Term

A well-stocked GFCF pantry makes it easier to maintain the diet without frequent shopping trips. Staples to include are gluten-free flours (like almond, coconut, and rice flour), plant-based milks (almond, coconut, oat milk), legumes, grains like quinoa and brown rice, nut butters, and a variety of herbs and spices. Investing in high-quality pantry items helps enhance meal variety and flavor.

Organizing the pantry by grouping similar items together—such as gluten-free baking ingredients, snacks, and meal bases—saves time and makes meal prep more efficient. Rotating items and checking expiration dates periodically ensures ingredients remain fresh.

Time-Saving Cooking Strategies

For busy parents, maintaining a GFCF diet can be challenging. Time-saving strategies like meal prepping and batch cooking are essential. Set aside time each week to prepare larger portions of staple foods, such as quinoa, grilled chicken, and steamed vegetables. These can be stored in the refrigerator or freezer and combined in different ways for quick meals throughout the week.

Utilizing slow cookers and instant pots can also make meal preparation easier. GFCF-friendly soups, stews, and casseroles can be prepared with minimal hands-on time and yield leftovers that last for days. Planning for leftovers and creating new meals from them, such as turning roasted chicken into chicken salad, reduces food waste and saves effort.

Dealing with Changing Preferences and Picky Eating

As children grow, their tastes and food preferences can change. This can pose challenges, especially if your child becomes selective or goes through a picky eating phase. Continue to offer a variety of foods without pressuring them to eat everything. The "one-bite rule" can be an effective way to encourage tasting new foods without overwhelming them. Even children without dietary restrictions can be picky eaters at times. As a mother, I've experienced firsthand how challenging it can be when my son suddenly decides he only wants to eat fish fingers one week and potatoes the next. I know how difficult it can be to accommodate these sudden changes in preference.

Experimenting with textures, flavors, and preparation methods can help keep meals appealing. For instance, if your child dislikes raw carrots, try roasting them with a drizzle of olive oil and a sprinkle of cinnamon for a different taste and texture. Integrating dips and sauces, such as dairy-free hummus or guacamole, can also make raw vegetables or plain foods more enticing.

Community and Support

Maintaining a GFCF diet is easier when you have a supportive community. Connect with other parents who follow a similar diet for recipe ideas, tips, and encouragement. Online forums, social media groups, and local support groups can be invaluable sources of information and shared experiences. Consider attending workshops or cooking classes that focus on GFCF recipes and nutrition to expand your meal repertoire and learn new skills.

Adapting the GFCF Diet for Special Situations

Special situations, such as vacations, school trips, and sleepovers, can present unique challenges. Preparing for these events with a proactive approach helps maintain consistency. Pack travel-friendly GFCF snacks like rice cakes, dried fruit, gluten-free granola bars, and nut mixes. For longer trips, research grocery stores and restaurants at your destination that offer GFCF options.

Communicate with teachers, caregivers, and the parents of your child's friends to ensure they understand the dietary needs. Share tips and provide GFCF-friendly snacks or meals that your child can eat at school or during outings. Planning ahead not only protects your child's health but also helps them feel included and comfortable in different settings.

Balancing Cost and Nutrition

Managing the cost of maintaining a GFCF diet can be challenging, but there are ways to make it more affordable. Purchasing items like gluten-free flours, grains, and legumes in bulk can help reduce expenses. Shopping for seasonal produce not only supports better pricing but also provides peak nutritional value.

Making GFCF staples at home can be both cost-effective and healthier. Homemade gluten-free bread, muffins, and snacks often cost less and allow you to control the ingredients, avoiding additives and preservatives. Prioritizing nutrient-dense, budget-friendly foods like rice, beans, and in-season vegetables ensures that your child's diet remains balanced and affordable.

Encouraging Independence

As children grow older, teaching them to take more responsibility for their diet helps them become more independent and confident in managing their dietary needs. Involve older children and teens in grocery shopping and meal prep. Show them how to read food labels for hidden sources of gluten and casein, and teach them basic cooking skills so they can prepare simple GFCF meals and snacks.

Developing these skills empowers them to make informed food choices, especially as they become more social and participate in activities where parents may not be present to monitor their diet. This independence helps them take ownership of their health and feel more in control.

Final Thoughts

Maintaining and adapting a GFCF diet as a long-term lifestyle requires flexibility, creativity, and support. By building a strong foundation with time-saving strategies, varied meal plans, and an organized pantry, parents can create a sustainable approach that grows with their child's needs. Engaging children in the process, connecting with a supportive community, and preparing for special situations all contribute to a successful, balanced GFCF diet that supports health and well-being at every stage of growth.

In the next chapter, we will explore how to handle challenges that arise when following a GFCF diet, including social situations, unplanned events, and setbacks, and how to navigate them with confidence and resilience.

CHAPTER 8: Handling Challenges and Setbacks in a GFCF Diet

Maintaining a GFCF (gluten-free, casein-free) diet for your child can present various challenges, from social situations to unexpected events and setbacks. Navigating these moments with confidence and resilience is key to ensuring long-term success and emotional well-being for both you and your child. This chapter will explore practical strategies for managing social gatherings, dealing with un-planned events, overcoming setbacks, and supporting your child in building self-advocacy and confidence.

Dealing with Social Situations

One of the most common challenges parents face when maintain-ing a GFCF diet is managing social situations like birthday parties, playdates, and family gatherings. These events often feature foods that may not align with your child's dietary needs, but with careful planning, your child can still fully participate and enjoy the occasion.

Reach out to the host or other parents before the event to discuss your child's dietary needs. Most people are understanding and will-ing to accommodate dietary restrictions when they are informed ahead of time. Share simple suggestions or offer to bring a GFCF dish that everyone can enjoy. Bring GFCF-friendly snacks or meals for your child to ensure they have something safe to eat. Pack items like gluten-free cupcakes for a birthday party or a small container of their favorite GFCF treats. This helps them feel included and reduces the temptation to eat something that may not be safe.Help your child understand what foods they should avoid and encourage them to ask questions if they are unsure about what's being served. Practice simple phrases with them, such as, "Is this gluten-free?" or "Does this have dairy in it?" Empowering your child to advocate for themselves builds confidence and reinforces healthy habits.

Life is full of unexpected events, from last-minute playdates to impromptu family outings. It's essential to be prepared for these moments so your child can maintain their diet even when plans change suddenly. Having a stash of GFCF-friendly snacks at home, in the car, or in your bag can make a significant difference. Granola bars, rice cakes, dried fruit, and nuts (if not allergic) are easy to pack and can be a lifesaver when you're on the go. As your child grows older, teaching them how to make safe choices independently is crucial. Explain which types of foods are usually safe (e.g., plain fruits and vegetables) and what to avoid. This helps them feel secure when they are in situations where you may not be present.

Navigating Peer Pressure and Questions
Children, especially as they grow older, may face questions or pressure from their peers about their dietary restrictions. This can lead to feelings of exclusion or embarrassment if not managed with care. Help your child develop simple explanations they can use when friends ask about their diet. Phrases like, "I eat this way to help my body feel better," or "I have to avoid certain foods so I stay healthy," can be empowering and clear.

Remind your child that having dietary restrictions doesn't make them different in a negative way; it simply means their body has specific needs. Highlight how many other people have dietary restrictions and that being mindful of their health is something to be proud of. Accidental consumption of gluten or casein can happen despite best efforts. When this occurs, it's important to stay calm and focus on

managing the situation effectively. If your child accidentally eats something they shouldn't reassure them that mistakes happen and they are not at fault. Create a plan for how to handle symptoms, such as keeping them hydrated, providing rest, and monitoring their condition. Having a designated comfort routine in place can help reduce anxiety.

Use setbacks as learning opportunities. Reflect on what led to the situation and discuss what can be done differently next time. This could involve reviewing how to read labels more carefully, double-checking with restaurant staff, or preparing better for future outings.

Adjusting After Challenges

It's natural to feel frustrated or disappointed after a dietary lapse, but focusing on moving forward is essential. Encourage your child to approach these moments with a positive mindset. Reinforce that maintaining a GFCF diet is a journey and that perfection isn't the goal. Emphasize the progress your child has made and celebrate their successes, no matter how small. This helps them maintain motivation and a healthy attitude toward their diet. After a setback, gently guide your child back into their regular eating routine. Returning to familiar and safe foods can help restore their sense of security and confidence.

Sticking to a GFCF diet can sometimes cause feelings of exclusion or frustration, particularly during social events or when dining out. Supporting your child's emotional well-being is crucial for maintaining a positive relationship with food. Ensure that your child feels included during celebrations by preparing GFCF-friendly versions of popular party foods. This can make a big difference in helping them feel part of the event. For example, bring GFCF cupcakes or cookies to parties or make GFCF pizza for family movie night. Acknowledge any feelings of frustration or sadness your child may have about their dietary restrictions. Encourage open conversations and reassure them that their feelings are valid. Share stories of others who have managed similar challenges to show that they're not alone.

Collaborating with Schools and Caregivers

Maintaining a GFCF diet requires the support of everyone involved in your child's life, including teachers, caregivers, and extended family.

Discuss your child's dietary needs with teachers and caregivers to ensure they understand the importance of following the GFCF diet. Provide clear instructions and suggest safe snacks or meals they can offer your child. Consider creating a simple care plan that outlines what your child can and cannot eat. Sending your child to school or activities with GFCF meals and snacks can prevent confusion and reduce the risk of accidental consumption. Labeling their lunchbox and containers can make it easier for caregivers to manage their diet.

As your child grows, teaching them to advocate for their dietary needs helps build independence and self-assurance. Show your child how to read food labels and recognize common ingredients that contain gluten or casein. Practice ordering food at restaurants to- gether, so they feel confident asking questions about menu items and food preparation. Role-playing different scenarios can prepare your child for real-life situations. Practice how they can politely de- cline food that doesn't meet their dietary requirements or ask ques- tions about food ingredients at social events.

Maintaining motivation can be challenging, especially when your child faces repeated setbacks or moments of frustration. Remind your child of the benefits they experience from following a GFCF diet, such as feeling healthier or more energetic. Keeping a "success journal" where you document moments of progress and accom- plishments can help reinforce the positive impact of the diet. Setting achievable, short-term goals can keep your child motivated. For in- stance, trying one new GFCF recipe each week or making a GFCF treat together can bring excitement to the routine.

Using Resources for Support

There are many tools and resources available to support a GFCF lifestyle. Utilize mobile apps that help identify gluten-free and ca- sein-free products, and follow online recipe blogs for fresh meal ideas. Joining a support group, either online or in person, can provide a sense of community and shared experience.

Final Thoughts

Challenges and setbacks are part of any journey, including maintaining a GFCF diet. By preparing for social situations, managing unplanned events, supporting emotional well-being, and teaching advocacy skills, you can help your child navigate obstacles with resilience and confidence. Your support and encouragement will empower them to stick to their diet and feel secure in their food choices, building a foundation for lifelong health and well-being. In the next chapter, we will discuss how to celebrate successes and create positive milestones that reinforce your child's commitment to their GFCF diet.

CHAPTER 9: Involving Your Child: Making Dietary Changes a Team Effort

Transitioning to a new diet can be daunting for any family, but it is especially significant for children who may be attached to certain foods and routines. Involving your child in the process can make all the difference, turning what might seem like a difficult change into an empowering and engaging journey. When children have an active role in making decisions about their diet, they are more likely to embrace new foods and be enthusiastic participants.

Involving your child in their dietary journey helps them develop a sense of responsibility and ownership over their food choices. This involvement not only promotes a willingness to try new foods but also encourages them to develop life skills and a positive relationship with nutrition. The goal is to create an environment where your child feels safe, engaged, and excited about making healthy choices.

Making Meal Planning a Collaborative Effort

One of the most effective ways to get your child excited about their diet is to involve them in planning meals. Sit down together to plan the week's menu, browsing cookbooks or online recipes that fit the GFCF guidelines. Allow your child to choose a few meals that they're eager to try. This process not only makes them feel heard but also helps them take pride in their choices. You might find that this collaborative planning sparks conversations about what ingredients they're curious about or dishes they've heard about from friends.

When it's time for grocery shopping, bring your child along. Turn the outing into an educational activity by showing them how to read labels and identify GFCF-friendly ingredients. Encourage them to help pick out fruits, vegetables, and other items. These simple acts teach them about making informed food choices and create an engaging experience. Use this opportunity to talk about where food comes from and why certain foods are better choices for them.

Getting Hands-On in the Kitchen

Cooking can be a fun and interactive way to involve your child in their diet. Start with simple tasks like washing vegetables, stirring ingredients, or measuring out portions. These activities help build confidence and familiarity with food preparation. Older children can help with more complex tasks like cracking eggs, mixing batters, or using blenders with supervision. These experiences not only empower them but also teach valuable life skills, such as following instructions, understanding food safety, and basic math through measuring.

Create opportunities for your child to design their own GFCF recipes or experiment with flavors. For instance, let them mix dairy-free yogurt with different fruits and toppings or come up with a custom sandwich filling. This creative freedom can transform the kitchen into a space of discovery and fun. You can even set aside one day a week for them to be the "head chef" and choose the menu for the evening, with your guidance.

Making Mealtime Fun with Themed Days

Turning meal prep into a special event can boost excitement about trying new dishes. Have themed cooking days like "Taco Tuesday," where your child can assemble their own gluten-free tacos with an array of toppings, or "Smoothie Sunday," where they choose fruits and mix-ins to create a dairy-free smoothie. These themed days turn food preparation into a shared activity, creating positive associations with their diet. You could expand this idea by incorporating global food days, such as "Italian Night" with gluten-free pasta or "Asian Fusion" with rice noodles and stir-fried vegetables. This introduces your child to different cuisines while staying within dietary guidelines.

Teaching Nutrition in a Kid-Friendly Way

Helping your child understand why their diet matters can deepen their commitment to the change. Use age-appropriate methods to explain the importance of healthy eating. You can create a food rainbow chart, showing them how different-colored fruits and vegetables provide essential nutrients. Encourage them to track how many colors they eat each day, making it a fun challenge.

Stories and analogies are also effective. You might tell them, "Eating vegetables gives you superhero energy," or explain that "protein helps build strong muscles like building blocks." Reinforce these ideas with practical examples: show them how choosing a snack like an apple and almond butter keeps them energized longer than a sugary treat. This reinforces that food choices affect how they feel and play. If your child enjoys screen time, watch kid-friendly cooking shows together. These shows can inspire them and make learning about food engaging.

Managing Resistance and Picky Eating

Introducing new foods can lead to resistance, especially for children with sensory sensitivities or strong food preferences. Patience and creativity are key. Encourage your child to take just one bite of a new food without pressure to eat more if they don't want to. Over time, this simple practice can build comfort with unfamiliar foods.

Turning the process into a game can also be helpful. Create a food adventure where they earn points or small rewards for trying something new. Serve familiar foods with small twists, like adding cinnamon to gluten-free pancakes or blending a new fruit into their favorite dairy-free yogurt. Try presenting new foods in fun and appealing ways, such as cutting them into interesting shapes or using small, colorful plates. The visual appeal can make new foods less intimidating

Building Routine and Consistency

Consistency helps children feel secure. Establish regular mealtimes and snacks to create a sense of routine. A calm eating environment without screens or loud distractions can make mealtimes more enjoyable and help your child focus on their food. When possible, eat meals together as a family. Seeing parents and siblings enjoying the same foods sets a positive example and encourages your child to follow suit.

Incorporating food routines into your day can also be a part of building a larger sense of security. For example, starting each day with a shared breakfast ritual or ending it with a simple dessert ritual using GFCF options can make dietary changes feel more like part of family life than an imposed rule.

Celebrating Achievements

Positive reinforcement is essential in fostering confidence. Celebrate your child's efforts, whether it's trying a new dish, helping in the kitchen, or making healthy choices on their own. Consider keeping a food adventure journal where they can write or draw about new foods they've tried and what they liked or didn't like. This journal can become a cherished keepsake that tracks their growth and the progress of their food journey. Hosting occasional "taste test" nights as a family can also be fun. Sample a few new GFCF dishes and share opinions, making the experience social and relaxed.

Create moments of celebration that aren't just about food. For example, if your child tries a new dish, reward them with an extra story at bedtime, a trip to the park, or a fun craft project. This reinforces that food exploration is a positive and enjoyable part of their life.

Supporting Their Emotional Connection with Food

Dietary changes can be a source of stress, so it's important to remind your child that their choices are about feeling their best and staying healthy. Reinforce a positive narrative, such as, "This food helps your body grow strong," or, "We're doing this to help you have more energy to play." This approach helps build a healthy relationship with food that extends beyond dietary restrictions.

If your child experiences setbacks, like disliking a new food or missing an old favorite, acknowledge their feelings. Saying something like, "I know you miss that, and that's okay. Let's find something new that you like just as much," helps validate their emotions while steering them toward positive solutions.

Encouraging Long-Term Interest

Maintaining your child's involvement as they grow can help sustain their interest in making healthy food choices. As they become more independent, teach them how to make simple GFCF meals themselves, fostering a sense of pride and self-reliance. Encourage them to take ownership of packing their own snacks for school or preparing their lunch, guiding them as needed.

Consider introducing them to food journaling as they grow older. They can document what they eat, how it makes them feel, and any new recipes they'd like to try. This empowers them to be proactive about their diet and can deepen their understanding of nutrition.

Involving your child in their GFCF diet can turn what might initially seem challenging into a shared adventure. These experiences empower them, make the process smoother for you, and instill lifelong skills that promote health and well-being. In the next chapter, we'll discuss how to track and measure improvements, observe changes over time, and understand the impact of the GFCF diet. This knowledge will equip you to make informed choices that continue supporting your child's growth and happiness.

CHAPTER 10: Celebrating Milestones and Positive Reinforcement in a GFCF Diet

Maintaining a GFCF (gluten-free, casein-free) diet is an ongoing journey that comes with challenges and victories. Recognizing and celebrating milestones along the way can have a profound impact on your child's relationship with food and their motivation to stick to their dietary needs. This chapter will explore ways to celebrate achievements, create positive reinforcement, and build a supportive environment that encourages your child to embrace their GFCF diet with confidence.

Recognizing and Celebrating Achievements

Every step your child takes toward maintaining their GFCF diet is worth acknowledging. Whether they've successfully navigated a social event without straying from their diet, tried a new GFCF dish, or confidently explained their dietary needs to someone, these moments represent significant achievements. Recognizing these accomplishments helps build self-esteem and reinforces positive behavior.

Celebrating achievements doesn't need to be extravagant; simple gestures like verbal praise or an enthusiastic high-five can be powerful motivators. Let your child know that their efforts are seen and appreciated, reinforcing their confidence and dedication.

Ways to Celebrate Milestones

There are many ways to celebrate dietary milestones that will make your child feel proud and motivated. Here are a few ideas:

- Special Family Meals: Plan a family dinner that features your child's favorite GFCF dishes. Let them choose the menu and involve them in preparing the meal.

- Homemade GFCF Treats: Surprise your child with homemade GFCF cupcakes, cookies, or a special dessert to mark a milestone, such as a month of successfully following their diet or trying a new food.

- Small Celebrations: Host a mini celebration at home with family and close friends. This could be for special occasions like birthdays or to recognize a specific achievement, like eating a full meal at a party without dietary mishaps.

Creating Reward Systems

A structured reward system can encourage positive behavior and help children stay motivated. Rewards don't need to be food-related; in fact, using non-food rewards can reinforce the idea that success and celebration aren't solely tied to eating. Examples include:

- Stickers or Reward Charts: Create a chart where your child earns a sticker or star for each goal achieved, such as trying a new GFCF food or packing their GFCF lunch.

- Small Prizes: Offer small toys, books, or art supplies as rewards for reaching dietary milestones.

- Extra Playtime: Allow additional time for a favorite activity, like playing at the park or having a movie night, as a way to celebrate their success.

These types of rewards help children build a positive association with their diet and reinforce that their efforts are worth celebrating

Building a Positive Relationship with Food

Fostering a positive relationship with food is vital for your child's long-term health and well-being. Encourage your child to see food as an enjoyable and nourishing part of life, even with dietary re-strictions. Here's how to help:

- Involve Them in the Kitchen: Let your child help with meal prep-aration. They can wash vegetables, stir batter, or choose ingredients for their meal. Participating in the process increases their excitement about trying new foods and makes them feel invested in their diet.

- Celebrate Curiosity: Encourage your child to explore new GFCF recipes and foods. Praise their willingness to try something new, even if they don't end up liking it. The act of exploration itself is worth celebrating.

- Make Mealtimes Fun: Use creative presentations and themes for meals, such as "Rainbow Night" where every dish includes different colored vegetables or "DIY Taco Night" with GFCF taco shells and toppings.

Celebrating Non-Food Achievements

It's important to broaden the scope of the celebration to include non-food-related achievements. This approach helps shift the focus from food itself to overall progress and effort. Examples of non-food achievements could include:

- Successfully Explaining Their Diet: If your child speaks up about their dietary needs at a social event or with friends, celebrate this step toward self-advocacy.

- Participating in Meal Prep: Recognize when your child takes the initiative to help make a GFCF meal or comes up with their own recipe ideas.

- Showing Resilience: Applaud moments when your child handles a challenging situation with grace, such as declining non-GFCF food at a party.

Recognizing Efforts, Not Just Outcomes

It's essential to recognize and celebrate your child's efforts, even when things don't go perfectly. Emphasizing effort over perfection helps foster resilience and encourages them to keep trying. If your child tastes a new GFCF dish but doesn't enjoy it, praise them for being brave enough to try. This approach reduces pressure and builds a positive outlook on their dietary journey.

Incorporating Celebrations into Daily Life

Celebrating achievements doesn't have to be limited to special occasions. Simple daily acknowledgments can go a long way in re-inforcing positive behavior. Compliment your child when they make a good dietary decision or express pride when they help with meal prep. These small, daily gestures create an environment where your child feels consistently supported and motivated.

Family Involvement in Celebrations

When the whole family participates in recognizing milestones, it strengthens the sense of support and community around the GFCF diet. Plan activities that everyone can enjoy, such as a family game night with GFCF snacks or a picnic featuring GFCF sandwiches and treats. Family involvement shows your child that their efforts are valued and shared by those they love.

Special GFCF Recipes for Celebratory Occasions

Including GFCF treats for special occasions ensures your child feels included and can fully participate in celebrations. GFCF birthday cakes, cupcakes, and cookies can be just as delicious and fun as their traditional counterparts. Experiment with recipes that are easy to make and customize them with your child's favorite flavors and dec-orations. This reinforces that a GFCF diet can still be full of tasty, celebratory foods.

Keeping a Milestone Journal

Encourage your child to keep a milestone journal where they can document their achievements and reflect on their progress. This journal can include moments like trying a new GFCF dish, staying committed to their diet during a difficult situation, or successfully explaining their dietary needs to a friend. Reviewing these entries can be an uplifting reminder of how far they've come and inspire them to continue.

Final Thoughts

Celebrating milestones and creating positive reinforcement is an essential part of maintaining a GFCF diet and fostering a healthy relationship with food. By recognizing achievements, involving the whole family in celebrations, and focusing on effort over perfection, you can support your child in their dietary journey with joy and encouragement. These practices help build confidence and resilience, making it easier for your child to embrace their diet as a positive and integral part of their life. In the next chapter, we'll explore how to maintain balance and adapt the GFCF diet to fit a growing and changing lifestyle, ensuring long-term success and well-being.

CHAPTER 11: Maintaining Balance and Adapting the GFCF Diet as Your Child Grows

As your child grows, their dietary needs and lifestyle will evolve, presenting new opportunities and challenges in maintaining a balanced GFCF (gluten-free, casein-free) diet. This chapter explores how to adapt the GFCF diet to meet changing nutritional requirements, support new activities and social dynamics, and promote independence and resilience. By understanding how to balance nutritional needs and lifestyle changes, parents can help their children continue thriving on a GFCF diet at every stage of development.

Adjusting the GFCF Diet for Growth and Development
Children's bodies undergo significant changes as they grow, especially during adolescence when growth spurts and hormonal changes create increased nutritional demands. These physical changes can affect energy levels, metabolism, and overall dietary needs, making it essential for parents to adjust the GFCF diet accordingly.

To meet these heightened energy requirements, ensure that your child's diet is rich in nutrient-dense foods. This means focusing on high-quality proteins such as eggs, fish, lean meats, beans, and fortified plant-based alternatives. These foods provide the essential amino acids necessary for muscle development and repair. Pair proteins with complex carbohydrates like sweet potatoes, brown rice, and gluten-free oats to provide sustained energy throughout the day. Healthy fats from sources like avocados, olive oil, and nuts are also essential for brain development and hormone regulation.

Adolescents, in particular, need more calcium and vitamin D to support bone health. Since dairy is excluded from a GFCF diet, parents need to find suitable alternatives. Fortified plant-based milks such as almond, soy, or oat milk can be excellent sources of calcium and vitamin D. Incorporate leafy greens, broccoli, and calcium-rich fish like canned salmon with bones into their meals. If needed, consult a healthcare provider about supplementing these nutrients to ensure optimal intake. A dietitian who specializes in GFCF diets can help assess whether your child's diet is meeting their nutritional needs and recommend any necessary adjustments or supplements.

Incorporating Cultural and Social Food Traditions

As children grow and develop socially, they may become more interested in cultural or traditional foods that their peers enjoy. Incorporating these traditions into a GFCF diet can help them feel more connected and included. Research and adapt popular cultural dishes to be GFCF-friendly. For example, gluten-free and dairy-free versions of common foods like pizza, tacos, sushi, or pasta dishes can be made at home with simple substitutions.

Discuss how holidays, celebrations, and family gatherings often center around specific dishes that may traditionally contain gluten or dairy. Work with your child to create GFCF versions of these beloved recipes, like gluten-free holiday cookies, dairy-free mac and cheese, or a GFCF stuffing for Thanksgiving. This not only allows them to participate in shared cultural experiences but also teaches them valuable cooking skills.

Navigating Food Trends and Fads

Teenagers and young adults are particularly susceptible to food trends and fads that promise health benefits or align with popular diets. It's important to help your child differentiate between trends that may benefit their GFCF lifestyle and those that could be potentially harmful or unnecessary. Discussing food trends openly, such as keto, paleo, or plant-based diets, provides an opportunity to explain their compatibility with GFCF eating and whether they meet their individual nutritional needs.

Encourage your child to research and critically assess any new diet or food trend they're interested in. This empowers them to make informed decisions and understand the importance of balanced nutrition over following trends. Sharing how to read scientific articles or consult reliable sources like registered dietitians can be a valuable part of this process.

Balancing Nutritional Needs with Lifestyle Changes

As children grow older, their activities often expand to include sports, dance, or other extracurricular pursuits that require additional energy and nutritional support. Adapting the GFCF diet to align with these activities helps maintain their performance and overall well-being. Balanced meals that include carbohydrates for immediate energy, proteins for muscle repair, and healthy fats for sustained energy release are crucial. For example, a breakfast of gluten-free toast with avocado and a side of scrambled eggs can provide a balanced mix of macronutrients to start the day.

Snacks are another important part of an active child's diet. GFCF snacks such as granola bars made with oats and seeds, fruit and nut mixes, or dairy-free yogurt with gluten-free granola can be easily prepared and packed for on-the-go energy. Encourage your child to carry snacks with them during busy school days or sports events to keep their energy levels steady. Hydration is equally critical, especially for children who engage in physical activities. Teach them the importance of drinking water throughout the day and provide hydrating snacks like oranges, watermelon, and cucumber slices to help them stay refreshed.

Balancing nutritional needs also means being aware of the timing of meals. For children involved in after-school sports, an early, protein-rich dinner followed by a lighter snack post-practice can help with muscle recovery and maintaining energy levels. For instance, a meal of grilled chicken, quinoa, and steamed vegetables provides protein and complex carbohydrates, while a post-activity snack of a banana with almond butter can replenish energy without being too heavy.

Incorporating New Foods and Expanding the Diet

As children grow, their tastes and preferences evolve. What they loved to eat as young children might not appeal to them as adolescents, and vice versa. Keeping the GFCF diet interesting and varied is key to ensuring that they continue to enjoy their meals and get a broad range of nutrients. Gradually introduce new types of vegetables, grains, and proteins to keep their diet diverse. For example, if your child is accustomed to rice as their main grain, try introducing quinoa, millet, or buckwheat for added variety and nutrition. Incorporating these foods into familiar dishes, like using quinoa in place of rice in stir-fries or adding millet to soups, can make new ingredients more approachable.

Encourage your child to experiment with different spices and seasonings to create flavors they enjoy. Allow them to be involved in choosing spices and seasoning blends for their meals. This involvement not only increases their interest in food but also teaches them about different flavor profiles and nutrition. For instance, spices like turmeric, cumin, and paprika can add depth to dishes and come with additional health benefits, such as anti-inflammatory properties.

Adding fermented foods such as kimchi, sauerkraut, and dairy-free yogurts with probiotics can also support gut health, which is crucial for nutrient absorption and overall well-being. Introducing your child to these foods early on can help them develop a palate for complex flavors and teach them about the importance of a balanced gut microbiome.

Supporting Independence in Food Preparation

Transitioning to cooking more complex meals can be a rewarding and confidence-building experience for teens. Encourage them to expand their cooking skills by exploring GFCF recipes that involve different cooking techniques, such as roasting, sautéing, or using an air fryer. Start with themed cooking nights at home where they can choose a new recipe, shop for ingredients, and prepare the meal with your guidance. This not only teaches them to cook but also shows them that maintaining a GFCF diet doesn't mean sacrificing variety or flavor.

Provide resources like online cooking tutorials, GFCF-focused YouTube channels, and interactive cooking classes. If possible, enroll them in community cooking workshops that cater to dietary restrictions or host small group sessions with friends where they can cook and learn together.

Teaching Healthy Eating Habits

Developing healthy eating habits is essential as children transition into adolescence and begin making more independent food choices. Teaching them about portion control and balanced meal composition can empower them to make informed decisions when choosing what to eat. Simple guidelines, such as visualizing a plate divided into halves and quarters—half vegetables, one quarter protein, and one quarter carbohydrates—can help them understand what a balanced meal looks like. For instance, a plate with grilled fish, steamed broccoli, and roasted sweet potatoes fits this guideline and offers a variety of nutrients.

Discussing the importance of variety in their diet and explaining why each food group contributes to their overall health is also important. Conversations about nutrition should be framed in an encouraging and non-restrictive way, emphasizing the benefits of eating well rather than focusing on limitations. This positive approach helps them associate healthy eating with self-care and long-term well-being.

Introduce them to the concept of intuitive eating, which involves listening to their body's hunger and fullness cues. This practice can prevent overeating and build a healthier relationship with food. Teaching them to recognize the difference between physical hunger and emotional eating can also help them develop self-awareness and make mindful food choices.

This might sound like repetition, but as nutritional gaps are related to this growing up, I have also included it in this chapter. As your child grows, ensuring that they get all the necessary vitamins and minerals is essential. Nutritional gaps can arise in any diet, but they are more likely with dietary restrictions like GFCF. Discuss specific nutrients that are often missed in a GFCF diet, such as B vitamins, iron, and omega-3 fatty acids. Guide your child on how to incorporate sources of these nutrients through foods like fortified cereals, leafy greens, fish, seeds, and legumes.

If supplementation is necessary, consult a healthcare professional who can recommend safe and effective options. Educating your child on why these nutrients are important and how to obtain them helps them take an active role in their health. Discuss the signs of nutritional deficiencies, such as fatigue, brittle hair and nails, or difficulty concentrating, and explain when it might be necessary to seek medical advice.

Final Thoughts

Adapting the GFCF diet as your child grows is a dynamic journey that requires patience, flexibility, and continued support. As your child enters different stages of life, their nutritional needs, social dynamics, and independence evolve, making it essential to adjust your approach accordingly. Whether it's increasing their understanding of balanced nutrition, teaching them how to prepare meals independently, or helping them navigate social situations with confidence, these changes are all part of helping your child thrive on a GFCF diet.

Throughout this process, remember that the goal is not just about adhering to dietary restrictions, but also about fostering a healthy relationship with food, empowering your child to make informed choices, and supporting their overall well-being. It's important to recognize and celebrate the small victories, whether that's mastering a new recipe, communicating dietary needs confidently, or simply feeling comfortable in their own skin.

The journey of maintaining a GFCF diet is not always easy, but by building resilience, offering emotional support, and staying informed, you can create an environment where your child can grow, adapt, and succeed. Each family's experience will be unique, but with dedication and the right resources, you can help your child navigate the challenges that come with a GFCF lifestyle and set them up for long-term success.

Remember that you are not alone in this journey. Whether it's connecting with other parents, seeking professional guidance, or exploring new recipes together, there are many resources and support systems available to help you along the way. By continuing to adapt the diet to meet your child's changing needs and celebrating their progress, you can ensure that the GFCF diet remains a positive, empowering part of their life.

CHAPTER 12: Preparing for Major Transitions and Long-Term Success on a GFCF Diet

As your child grows and matures, their dietary needs, preferences, and lifestyle will evolve. Transitioning from childhood to adolescence and eventually into adulthood comes with new challenges, opportunities, and responsibilities. This chapter will explore how to maintain a GFCF (gluten-free, casein-free) diet through these major life transitions, ensure long-term success, and instill lifelong habits that support overall health and well-being.

Transitioning from Childhood to Adolescence

Adolescence brings significant physical, emotional, and social changes. Increased independence, greater peer influence, and evolving self-identity are key aspects of this stage. Navigating these changes while maintaining a GFCF diet requires patience, understanding, and a shift in how parents support their child's dietary needs.

One of the most notable changes during adolescence is a greater desire for independence, including making their own food choices. To foster this independence while ensuring adherence to the GFCF diet, start by involving your teen more directly in meal planning and preparation. Teach them how to make balanced meals, read food labels, and identify safe GFCF options when dining out or at school.

Preparing for High School and College

High school and college present new challenges as teens and young adults are exposed to more social events, dining out with friends, and food options that may not align with their diet. To prepare them for these situations, focus on building strong advocacy and communication skills. Encourage them to feel confident in speaking up about their dietary needs, whether it's at a restaurant, a friend's house, or school cafeteria.

For college-bound teens, discuss how to navigate dining halls and dormitory food options. Many universities accommodate dietary restrictions, but it's important for your child to know how to advocate for themselves, ask questions, and seek out safe foods. Before moving to college, take time to explore options like meal prep services that offer GFCF meals, or how to stock a small dormitory kitchen with essential GFCF staples.

Building Lifelong Habits

Instilling habits that last into adulthood starts with consistent practice and education. Teach your child how to plan meals that are balanced and varied, emphasizing the importance of whole foods and nutrient diversity. Show them how to budget for groceries and make informed choices to keep a GFCF diet cost-effective and sustainable.

Learning to read ingredient labels and identifying hidden sources of gluten and casein should be second nature by this stage. Encourage your child to continue researching new GFCF-friendly products and recipes, reinforcing that their diet can evolve and include new foods.

Adapting to New Social and Academic Environments

Entering new social and academic environments can be intimidating for any child, especially one with dietary restrictions. Whether your child is joining a new sports team, participating in school events, or attending social gatherings, preparation is key. Teach them how to pack GFCF snacks and meals that travel well, so they always have a safe option on hand. Discuss how to handle situations where GFCF options may be limited and practice politely declining foods that don't meet their needs.

Encourage them to find supportive friends who respect and understand their dietary requirements. Having a peer group that values their health choices can reduce feelings of exclusion and reinforce positive dietary habits.

Handling Emotional and Social Pressures

Teenage years come with heightened social and emotional pressures. Your child may feel self-conscious about being different or frustrated with the limitations of their diet. Support their emotional well-being by fostering open conversations where they feel safe expressing their feelings. Acknowledge any frustrations or challenges they face and reassure them that their feelings are valid.

Provide positive coping strategies, such as journaling, mindfulness exercises, or joining a support group where they can share experiences with others who follow similar diets. Emphasize that their health and well-being come first, and making choices that support their diet is something to be proud of, not embarrassed about.

Maintaining Balance During Lifestyle Changes

Life transitions such as moving, starting a new school, or dealing with changing family dynamics can disrupt routines. Maintaining a GFCF diet during these times requires planning and flexibility. When possible, prepare for these changes by setting up a basic plan for meals and snacks that can be easily adjusted as needed.

Help your child re-establish routines once the transition is complete. This could include setting aside specific days for grocery shopping and meal prep or creating a go-to list of quick GFCF meals that don't require much preparation. Staying organized can make maintaining the diet feel more manageable during uncertain times.

Independence and Self-Advocacy

Teaching your teen or young adult how to advocate for their dietary needs is crucial as they start to navigate life more independently. Encourage them to practice discussing their dietary requirements in different settings, such as with friends, at restaurants, or in job interviews. Simple, clear explanations like, "I need to follow a gluten-free, dairy-free diet for my health" can help them feel confident in asserting their needs.

Role-playing different scenarios can be an effective way to build confidence. Practice situations such as ordering at a restaurant, explaining their diet to a new friend, or speaking up at work functions.

The more familiar these conversations become, the easier they will be to handle in real life.

Transitioning to Adulthood

Transitioning into adulthood means taking full ownership of dietary choices and overall health. Support your young adult by teaching them essential skills such as meal planning, grocery shopping, and cooking. Provide them with resources like GFCF cookbooks or reputable recipe sites that they can use to discover new dishes.

Budgeting is another critical aspect of managing a GFCF diet in adulthood. Help them understand how to prioritize purchases, find cost-effective GFCF products, and plan meals that are both nutritious and budget-friendly.

For young adults who are moving out or living with roommates, provide advice on how to manage shared kitchens and prevent cross-contamination. Encourage them to communicate their dietary needs openly and establish clear boundaries to maintain their health.

Continuing Professional Support

Even as children grow into teens and young adults, continued support from healthcare professionals is important. Encourage them to maintain regular check-ins with a doctor or dietitian familiar with GFCF diets to monitor their nutritional status and make any necessary adjustments. Professional guidance ensures they're meeting all their nutritional needs and can help them adapt their diet as their lifestyle evolves.

When searching for a new healthcare provider, look for professionals who have experience with dietary restrictions and who understand the complexities of a GFCF diet. This can provide valuable support and help them navigate changes in their health as they grow.

Staying Motivated Long-Term

Staying motivated to adhere to a GFCF diet can be challenging, especially over the long term. Encourage your child to set personal health goals, whether it's maintaining energy levels, improving digestion, or simply feeling their best. Joining support groups or online communities can encourage, share new GFCF recipes, and offer a sense of camaraderie.

Remind your child that staying informed and adapting as needed is part of the journey. Keeping up with new developments in GFCF products, restaurants, and dietary research can help them feel connected and inspired to continue their lifestyle.

Final Thoughts

Transitioning from childhood through adolescence and into adulthood on a GFCF diet requires adaptability, patience, and continuous support. By fostering independence, teaching advocacy skills, and reinforcing positive habits, parents can empower their children to manage their diet confidently. As they grow, balancing their nutritional needs with an active and changing lifestyle ensures they can continue to thrive. The key to long-term success lies in building a foundation of knowledge, resilience, and self-confidence that carries them into adulthood and beyond.

CHAPTER 13: Tips for Parents to Support Long-Term Success on a GFCF Diet

Supporting your child or young adult in maintaining a GFCF (gluten-free, casein-free) diet is an ongoing process that extends well beyond childhood. As they grow and their lifestyle, preferences, and challenges evolve, parents play a pivotal role in reinforcing healthy habits and encouraging resilience. This chapter provides detailed strategies for fostering independence, promoting a positive relationship with food, and ensuring that the GFCF diet becomes a sustainable part of their life.

Encouraging Lifelong Learning and Adaptation

The world of nutrition is ever-changing, with new research, products, and strategies continuously emerging. Instilling a mindset of lifelong learning in your child can help them adapt and make informed decisions throughout their life. Encourage your child to stay curious about their diet by exploring reputable online resources, joining workshops, and experimenting with new recipes. Parents can model this behavior by learning alongside their child—discovering new GFCF ingredients, trying different cooking techniques, and reading up on the latest studies related to gluten and casein sensitivity. This not only keeps their diet varied and exciting but also reinforces that managing their diet is a collaborative effort and part of their overall wellness journey.

Empowering Your Child to Take Ownership

Taking ownership of dietary habits is a vital step in fostering independence and self-confidence. Begin by gradually involving your child in all aspects of their diet. Teach them how to read and understand ingredient labels, emphasizing hidden sources of gluten and casein that might not be obvious. Take them on grocery shopping trips where they can select GFCF foods themselves, giving them the opportunity to learn which products fit their dietary needs.

Encourage meal planning by having them choose dishes for the week and helping them create balanced menus. Guide them through the process of preparing meals, starting with simpler dishes and progressing to more complex recipes as their confidence grows. The ability to cook nutritious GFCF meals independently is a valuable skill, especially as they transition to living more autonomously in high school, college, or adulthood.

Maintaining Flexibility and Openness

Maintaining a GFCF diet doesn't have to be rigid; in fact, flexibility is key to long-term success. Children and teens often change their food preferences as they grow, so being open to experimenting with new foods and adapting meals is important. Explore different cuisines that naturally align with a GFCF diet, such as Mediterranean, Asian, and Latin American dishes, to introduce a variety of flavors and ingredients. This can prevent dietary fatigue and make mealtimes more enjoyable.

Be open to trying new GFCF products that come to market. Many brands continually develop improved versions of gluten- and dairy-free foods, such as breads, pastas, and cheeses. Incorporating these products can add excitement and diversity to meals, making it easier to stick to the diet.

Fostering a Positive and Supportive Environment

A supportive home environment is fundamental for maintaining a positive outlook on dietary restrictions. Avoid framing the GFCF diet in negative terms like "can't have" or "restricted." Instead, emphasize the health benefits and delicious foods they can enjoy. Create a space where your child feels comfortable discussing their diet, sharing their successes, and expressing any challenges they face.

Celebrate even the small victories, like trying a new food or successfully managing their diet at a social event. Verbal encouragement, high-fives, or even small, non-food-related rewards can reinforce these achievements. Consistent positive reinforcement helps your child view their diet not as a limitation but as an empowering choice that supports their well-being.

Encouraging Social Inclusion

Social situations can be challenging when following a GFCF diet, but with preparation, they can be inclusive and enjoyable. Teach your child to bring GFCF-friendly snacks or dishes to share at parties or events so they don't feel excluded. This not only ensures they have something safe to eat but also showcases to others that GFCF foods can be just as tasty and satisfying.

When eating out, choose restaurants that offer gluten-free and dairy-free options. Review the menu beforehand, if possible, and teach your child how to ask questions about food preparation to confirm that dishes meet their dietary needs. Hosting gatherings at home with plenty of GFCF options can also help your child feel proud of their diet and demonstrate to friends and family that their meals can be enjoyed by everyone.

Developing Resilience and Problem-Solving Skills

Challenges related to maintaining a GFCF diet are inevitable, whether it's being offered food that isn't compliant at a party or navigating limited food options at an event. Preparing your child to handle these situations calmly and confidently is essential. Role-playing different scenarios helps them practice how to politely decline non-GFCF food or find alternative options.

Discuss backup plans they can use when faced with limited choices, such as opting for naturally GFCF foods like fruits, plain vegetables, and simple proteins, or carrying emergency snacks. Building problem-solving skills fosters resilience, giving your child the confidence to handle unexpected situations and maintain their diet.

Promoting Healthy Mindsets

A positive mindset toward their diet can greatly influence your child's adherence and motivation. Reinforce that their GFCF diet is a proactive choice that supports their health and helps them feel their best. Shift the focus from what they cannot have to what they can enjoy, and encourage them to think creatively about meals and snacks.

Highlight the benefits they experience from following their diet, such as increased energy, better digestion, or clearer skin. Remind them that everyone has unique dietary needs and that their diet is part of what makes them special. This mindset helps them feel empowered and less restricted, turning what could be seen as a limitation into a strength.

Setting Realistic Goals

Helping your child set realistic, achievable goals related to their diet can keep them engaged and motivated. Goals can range from trying one new GFCF recipe each week to preparing their own lunch for school or understanding how to read ingredient labels independently. Celebrate these milestones, no matter how small, to build confidence and show that progress is valued over perfection.

Setting long-term goals, such as mastering a set of GFCF recipes or successfully managing their diet at a social event without assistance, can give them something to work toward and feel proud of achieving.

Encouraging Peer Support

Finding peers who share similar dietary needs can provide valuable social support and reduce feelings of isolation. Encourage your child to join local or online groups focused on GFCF living, where they can exchange recipes, share tips, and discuss challenges. Having friends who understand and respect their dietary needs can be a powerful source of encouragement and make social situations easier to navigate.

Modeling Positive Behaviors as Parents

Children learn a lot from observing their parents. Show them that maintaining a GFCF diet is not only manageable but also beneficial. Involve yourself in meal planning, join them in trying new GFCF recipes, and demonstrate how to handle dietary challenges with a positive attitude. When your child sees you approach their diet calmly and confidently, they are more likely to adopt those behaviors themselves.

Handle any challenges or slip-ups with grace. If a mistake happens, such as accidentally consuming a non-GFCF food, model how to react calmly and refocus on moving forward. This teaches them that setbacks are a normal part of any process and can be managed without stress or frustration.

Reviewing and Reevaluating the Diet Regularly

As children grow, their nutritional needs and preferences change. Regularly reviewing the GFCF diet with a healthcare provider or dietitian helps ensure that it continues to meet their needs. These check-ins provide opportunities to discuss potential dietary adjustments, whether it's incorporating more nutrient-dense foods, adding supplements, or exploring new GFCF products that enhance their diet.

This proactive approach reassures your child that their health is a priority and encourages them to view their diet as adaptable, not static. It reinforces that they have control over their dietary choices and that adjustments can be made to support their changing life-style.

Celebrating Long-Term Successes

Long-term adherence to a GFCF diet is an accomplishment worth celebrating. Mark yearly milestones with a special meal, a family outing, or a small party with friends that includes their favorite GFCF foods. These celebrations reinforce the positive impact of the diet and serve as a reminder of their resilience and dedication.

Encourage your child to look back at how far they've come, acknowledging challenges they've overcome and the successes they've experienced. Reflecting on these moments helps them feel proud of their journey and strengthens their commitment to maintaining their diet in the future.

Final Thoughts

Supporting a child through their GFCF journey as they grow into a teen and young adult is a continuous process that requires patience, adaptability, and unwavering support. By empowering them to take ownership of their diet, fostering a positive environment, and encouraging resilience, parents can set the foundation for lifelong health and confidence. Through open communication, positive reinforcement, and a proactive approach, the GFCF diet can become an integral and beneficial part of their life, paving the way for well-being and success into adulthood.

CHAPTER 14: Preparing for the Future and Embracing Lifelong GFCF Success

As your child grows into adulthood, maintaining a GFCF (gluten-free, casein-free) diet becomes part of a larger journey of health and self-management. While childhood and adolescence are times when parents play a significant role in guiding and supporting dietary habits, adulthood brings increased independence and the responsibility of managing one's own health. This chapter will discuss how to prepare your child for a future where they confidently navigate their GFCF diet, sustain lifelong habits, and approach their health proactively.

Embracing Independence and Personal Responsibility

Transitioning from adolescence to adulthood is a critical period for developing personal responsibility in managing dietary needs. Helping your child embrace independence involves teaching them practical skills, such as budgeting for groceries, planning balanced meals, and cooking for themselves. These essential life skills empower them to make informed choices and maintain their dietary restrictions with confidence.

To prepare your child, start by creating a checklist that includes GFCF staples, meal ideas, and a variety of nutrient-dense foods. Teaching them how to plan their grocery trips ensures they select products that align with their dietary needs while balancing costs. Reinforce these skills by encouraging them to experiment with GFCF recipes on their own and manage their meal plans independently. Regular practice in the kitchen builds competence and familiarity, making cooking an enjoyable aspect of their self-care routine.

Cooking is not just a skill; it's a means of nurturing oneself. Encourage your child to see managing their GFCF diet as part of self-care, akin to regular exercise or maintaining good mental health practices. This view helps them appreciate the importance of their dietary choices and integrate them into their overall lifestyle.

Preparing for College and Independent Living

When your child prepares to leave home for college or independent living, they will need to feel confident managing their GFCF diet without direct parental support. Work with them to create a checklist of essentials for their new living space, such as a mini-fridge, small kitchen appliances, and airtight containers for storing food. Discuss basic cooking tools they might need, including a blender, cutting board, and microwave-safe dishes.

Review simple meal plans they can use as a starting point, and suggest building a collection of easy, go-to GFCF recipes. Recipes like stir-fry, gluten-free pasta with homemade sauce, or dairy-free smoothies can be made with minimal equipment and ingredients. Show them how to meal prep efficiently by cooking multiple servings at once to save time and reduce stress during busy school or workweeks.

Navigating college dining halls and local restaurants can be intimidating, so encourage them to communicate directly with dining staff to understand which options are safe. If possible, arrange a meeting or call with the campus dining services before the semester begins to discuss available GFCF options and any accommodations they may need.

Sustaining Healthy Habits Through Major Life Changes

Life is full of transitions, from moving out of the family home and starting college or a new job to building relationships and possibly starting a family of their own. These changes can disrupt routines, making it challenging to maintain a GFCF diet. Equip your child with strategies to adapt their diet during major life events, such as moving to a new city where familiar GFCF foods might not be readily available or adjusting to a new work schedule.

Teach them to plan ahead and research their new environment for GFCF-friendly stores, restaurants, and resources. Discuss the importance of creating meal plans that align with a busy schedule, and encourage them to find new support networks, whether through local meetups, online groups, or joining communities that share similar dietary needs.

Establishing Routines That Support a GFCF Lifestyle

Routines play an important role in maintaining dietary habits, especially during periods of transition like starting a new job or moving to a different city. Work with your child to establish daily and weekly routines that support a GFCF diet. These might include designating a specific day each week for grocery shopping, meal prepping, or trying a new recipe. Help them plan a balanced schedule that includes time for self-care, exercise, and relaxation, which can all support adherence to their diet and reduce stress.

Discuss how to manage their diet when life becomes hectic, such as during work projects, exams, or personal obligations. Teach them how to create a list of go-to meals that can be prepared quickly, like a GFCF smoothie bowl or a simple salad with pre-cooked protein and a dairy-free dressing. Having these routines and fallback options helps maintain consistency.

Building Confidence in New Settings

Starting a new chapter in life, such as attending college or working in a professional environment, requires confidence in advocating for one's dietary needs. Teach your young adult how to communicate effectively in new settings, whether it's talking to a roommate about shared kitchen spaces or explaining dietary restrictions to coworkers and supervisors. Role-play potential conversations to prepare them for questions or scenarios where they need to assert their needs confidently.

Encourage them to research dining options when traveling or attending events, and equip them with strategies for handling social gatherings where food may be central. This preparation empowers them to make informed choices and maintain their GFCF diet even in unfamiliar situations.

Developing Resilience and Coping Skills

Resilience is an essential skill for dealing with setbacks, such as accidentally consuming gluten or dairy. Teach your child that mistakes happen and that it's important to stay calm and know how to respond. If they experience symptoms, encourage them to have a plan in place, such as taking over-the-counter remedies or resting until they feel better.

Help them build coping mechanisms for emotional challenges related to dietary restrictions, such as feeling excluded or frustrated. Mindfulness practices, journaling, and relaxation techniques can help them manage stress and maintain a positive outlook. Remind them that dietary choices are part of a larger self-care strategy that supports their health and well-being.

Creating a Support System

Maintaining a GFCF diet can sometimes feel isolating, particularly in new environments where dietary restrictions may not be common. Encourage your child to build a network of friends, colleagues, or online communities that understand and support their dietary needs. This support system can provide emotional encouragement, share recipes and meal ideas, and help your child navigate challenges.

Supportive friends and mentors can make a significant difference, offering reassurance and a shared commitment to the diet. Encourage your child to reach out to peers who have similar dietary needs or who show an interest in learning about GFCF eating. Joining a GFCF group on social media or attending health-focused meetups can help them connect with others who understand their journey and can offer practical advice.

Building a Network of Health Professionals

Encourage your child to build a network of healthcare providers, including nutritionists, dietitians, and primary care doctors who are knowledgeable about dietary restrictions. These professionals can provide valuable insights and support as your child's needs evolve over time. Finding trusted experts who understand the GFCF lifestyle ensures that any health issues related to diet are addressed promptly and effectively.

Discuss the importance of annual or biannual check-ups to monitor health indicators that may be impacted by their diet, such as bone density, blood vitamin levels, and gut health. This proactive approach reinforces the idea that maintaining a GFCF diet is part of a comprehensive health strategy.

Managing Challenges in Adulthood

As adults, your child will encounter new challenges related to their diet, such as navigating restaurant menus during business meetings, participating in potlucks, or managing their diet while traveling internationally. Provide them with tips on how to research menus ahead of time, what questions to ask at restaurants, and how to advocate for themselves in social or professional situations.

Encourage them to travel with GFCF-friendly snacks, research international GFCF foods and ingredients, and learn how to communicate dietary restrictions in different languages if traveling abroad. These strategies will help them feel more confident and prepared for any situation that arises.

Staying Flexible and Open-Minded

Life will inevitably change, and with it, so may your child's approach to their diet. Encourage them to stay flexible and open-minded, recognizing that adjustments might be necessary over time. This could mean experimenting with new foods, changing meal routines, or reassessing their diet based on new research or life circumstances. Adapting to new situations with a positive outlook can make managing their diet less stressful and more integrated into their everyday life.

Being open to change does not mean disregarding their commitment to the GFCF diet, but rather understanding that living healthily is a dynamic process. Discuss times when it might be appropriate to consult a healthcare professional about dietary modifications, such as incorporating foods they once avoided or trying new GFCF products that offer more variety.

Staying Motivated and Embracing Health Beyond the Diet

Maintaining motivation for a GFCF diet can become more challenging as life grows busier and responsibilities multiply. Encourage your young adult to set health goals that go beyond dietary adherence, integrating their diet into a broader wellness routine. Regular exercise, mindfulness practices, and sufficient sleep contribute to their overall health and help maintain the motivation to follow a GFCF lifestyle.

Viewing their diet as part of a holistic approach to well-being helps them appreciate its benefits. Remind them to periodically reassess their diet and be open to adjustments based on changes in their health, lifestyle, or new research findings. For example, they may find new GFCF products or recipes that add variety to their meals, keeping their diet interesting and sustainable.

Encourage them to stay informed and curious, reading up on the latest GFCF research and new product offerings. Staying educated not only helps them make informed choices but also fosters a sense of control and empowerment.

Reflecting on Progress and Achievements

Reflection is an important part of embracing lifelong dietary habits. Encourage your child to take time to reflect on their progress, celebrating the milestones they achieve along the way. Whether it's successfully preparing a week's worth of GFCF meals, handling a challenging social event, or mastering a new recipe, acknowledging these achievements can boost their confidence and reinforce the importance of their efforts.

Suggest maintaining a journal where they can record positive experiences, new recipes they enjoyed, or any personal goals related to their diet and health. This reflective practice can be motivating and help them stay committed over the long term.

Empowering Them to Inspire Others

As they become more confident in their GFCF journey, encourage your child to share their experiences with others who might be starting out or struggling with their own dietary needs. They could write about their experiences, share recipes on social media, or participate in support groups. Inspiring others not only provides encouragement to those who are new to the lifestyle but also reinforces their own commitment and helps them recognize how far they've come.

Emphasize that being a role model doesn't require perfection but rather honesty and resilience. Sharing stories of overcoming challenges, adapting to new situations, and finding joy in their GFCF lifestyle can have a positive impact on both their journey and the community they reach.

Celebrating Their Journey

Acknowledging the journey from childhood to adulthood while adhering to a GFCF diet is essential for reinforcing their accomplishments. Celebrating milestones, whether big or small, helps boost confidence and maintain motivation. This could be as simple as mastering a new recipe, successfully managing their diet during a trip, or advocating for their needs at work or social events.

Encourage your young adult to document their journey, whether through journaling, sharing their experiences with friends, or participating in support groups. Reflecting on their growth and the challenges they've overcome can provide valuable motivation to continue prioritizing their health. Journaling, in particular, allows them to look back at how far they've come, reinforcing a sense of achievement and resilience.

Celebrating doesn't always need to be formal; it could be treating themselves to a new GFCF dish at a restaurant, hosting a gathering with friends to showcase their favorite recipes, or simply taking time to acknowledge their efforts and dedication.

Building a Healthy Relationship with Food

Developing a positive relationship with food is critical for sustaining long-term dietary habits. Emphasize that food is not only a necessity but also a source of nourishment, joy, and connection. Encourage your child to approach their diet with a mindset of abundance rather than restriction, focusing on the variety of foods they can enjoy and the health benefits they bring.

Exploring new cuisines and cooking with friends can be a fun way to keep meals exciting and engaging. Attending cooking classes that focus on GFCF recipes or experimenting with international dishes that are naturally gluten- and dairy-free can expand their culinary repertoire and make the diet feel less limiting. Creating positive experiences around food reinforces that a GFCF diet can be both enjoyable and fulfilling.

Help them learn to appreciate the flavors and textures of GFCF foods and find creative ways to replicate dishes they love using GFCF ingredients. Building a library of go-to recipes that are quick, easy, and satisfying ensures that they always have options they enjoy.

Maintaining Professional Support

Even as they grow older, encourage your young adult to continue seeking professional support when needed. Nutritionists, dietitians, and healthcare professionals can provide valuable guidance, particularly during major life transitions or if health concerns arise. Regular consultations with professionals who are knowledgeable about dietary restrictions can help them maintain a balanced diet, address potential nutritional gaps, and make informed adjustments to their eating habits.

Finding healthcare providers who are supportive and knowledgeable about GFCF needs ensures they receive comprehensive care that aligns with their lifestyle. It can also be beneficial to join workshops or seminars led by experts who can offer insights into maintaining a balanced diet and staying informed about new developments in GFCF nutrition.

Final Thoughts

Adapting a GFCF diet as your child grows into adulthood involves continuous learning, flexibility, and proactive support. By helping them build the skills to maintain their diet independently, navigate social and professional environments, and stay motivated, parents set their children up for lifelong health and well-being. Through preparation, open communication, and fostering resilience, you empower them to approach their GFCF diet as a positive, integrated part of their life. As they navigate adulthood, they'll carry with them the confidence, skills, and knowledge needed to thrive.

Chapter 15: Creating a GFCF-Friendly Kitchen and Home Environment

Creating a GFCF-friendly (gluten-free, casein-free) kitchen and home environment is essential for long-term success. This requires thoughtful organization, careful meal prep, and an understanding of how to prevent cross-contamination. Establishing these practices helps create a safe and supportive space that simplifies maintaining the diet for the whole family.

Setting up your kitchen to support GFCF living involves creating distinct areas and using dedicated tools. This can start with having specific shelves or cabinets for storing only GFCF foods. Labeling these areas can help prevent confusion and make it easy for everyone in the household to identify safe foods. Investing in separate utensils, cutting boards, and mixing bowls used exclusively for GFCF meal prep can make a significant difference in preventing cross-contamination. Color-coding these items is a helpful way to ensure that they are not accidentally used for non-GFCF foods. Regularly cleaning cooking surfaces is another essential practice. Wiping down counters and stovetops before preparing GFCF meals minimizes the risk of gluten or dairy particles contaminating the space.

For families who share kitchens with members who do not follow the GFCF diet, maintaining a safe cooking environment involves taking additional precautions. Labeling and dividing kitchen storage spaces, such as drawers and cabinets, can keep GFCF foods separate from others. Using separate appliances, like toasters, or toaster bags for dual use can help maintain safety. High-risk contamination points, such as communal butter dishes or condiment jars, should be avoided by using individually portioned containers or separately labeled versions for GFCF use.

Stocking a pantry with essential GFCF items is an important part of being prepared for meals and snacks. This could include basics like rice flour, gluten-free oats, and canned beans for budget-friendly options, as well as almond flour and chia seeds for more varied recipes. Including legumes, nuts, and dairy-free milk alternatives can add both nutrition and flexibility to meal planning. A well-organized pantry can be enhanced with clear containers and labels to make meal prep faster and more efficient. Keeping a seasonal rotation of pantry items, such as canned pumpkin puree in the fall or dried fruits in the summer, can ensure that ingredients stay fresh and align with available produce.

Meal prepping saves time and reduces stress, especially during busy weeks. Choose a day of the week to prepare and portion GFCF meals such as soups, casseroles, and baked goods. These can be stored in airtight containers in the refrigerator or freezer, making them quick to reheat when needed. Freezer storage tips include laying bags of soups flat for easy stacking and individually wrapping baked items to maintain freshness. Organizing the refrigerator with dedicated GFCF sections can further prevent accidental contamination and streamline the cooking process.

Reading labels effectively is crucial to maintaining a GFCF diet, as many products contain hidden sources of gluten and dairy. It's important to scan for allergen warnings, as labels will often indicate if a product contains wheat or milk. However, certain ingredients, like malt, modified food starch, and whey, may not be as obvious but still pose a risk. Familiarizing yourself with these potential hidden ingredients helps you make safer choices. Products labeled as "certified gluten-free" or "dairy-free" offer extra reassurance.

Certain kitchen tools and gadgets can simplify GFCF meal prep. A high-speed blender is invaluable for making smoothies, soups, and dairy-free ice cream, while a food processor is useful for making hummus and finely chopping ingredients. A bread machine with a gluten-free setting makes baking fresh bread at home easier, and an instant pot can speed up the cooking of grains and stews. Non-porous cutting boards made of silicone or glass are easy to sanitize and help prevent contamination, while air-tight containers keep GFCF ingredients fresh and safe. Color-coded utensils further ensure that everyone in the household can easily differentiate between GFCF items and those used for other foods. For those on a budget, affordable alternatives include reusable silicone mats for baking and manual hand mixers instead of electric ones.

A well-organized and maintained kitchen supports not only your child's dietary needs but also contributes to a smoother daily routine and peace of mind.

Kitchen Setup for GFCF Living

Creating a safe kitchen environment is crucial for preventing cross-contamination, which can occur when gluten or dairy comes into contact with GFCF food items or surfaces. Here's how to set up your kitchen for success:

1. Designate Specific Areas for GFCF Foods

Set aside specific shelves or cabinets for storing GFCF foods. This separation helps avoid confusion and accidental cross-contamination with non-GFCF items. Label these areas clearly for easy identification.

2. Use Dedicated Utensils and Cookware

Invest in separate cutting boards, baking sheets, toasters, and mixing bowls that are used exclusively for preparing GFCF foods. Color-coding these items can make it easier to remember which utensils are safe to use.

3. Clean Cooking Surfaces Thoroughly

Before preparing GFCF meals, wipe down counters, stovetops, and other surfaces with a damp cloth or disinfecting wipes. This simple step minimizes the risk of gluten or dairy particles contaminating the area.

4. Replace Common Kitchen Items

Swap out shared items like wooden spoons, cutting boards, and colanders, which can retain gluten particles even after washing. Opt for non-porous materials such as silicone or stainless steel, which are easier to clean thoroughly.

Stocking a GFCF Pantry

A well-stocked pantry ensures that you always have the essentials on hand for quick and nutritious GFCF meals. Here's what to include:

Essential GFCF Pantry Items:

- Gluten-Free Flours and Starches: Almond flour, coconut flour, rice flour, tapioca starch, and arrowroot powder for baking and cooking.

- Dairy-Free Milk Alternatives: Almond milk, coconut milk, oat milk, and soy milk for cooking, baking, and drinking.

- Grains: Quinoa, brown rice, millet, and gluten-free oats.

- Legumes and Beans: Chickpeas, lentils, black beans, and white beans for protein and fiber.

- Nuts and Seeds: Almonds, sunflower seeds, chia seeds, flaxseeds, and pumpkin seeds for snacks and meal additions.

- Dairy-Free Condiments: Coconut oil, olive oil, tahini, and nut butters.

- Snacks: GFCF crackers, popcorn, rice cakes, and dairy-free chips.

- Spices and Seasonings: Gluten-free labeled spices and seasoning mixes to flavor meals.

Tips for Organizing Your Pantry:

- Use clear containers to store flours, grains, and snacks. Label each container to avoid confusion.

- Group items by category (e.g., baking, snacks, grains) to make meal prep faster and more efficient.

- Keep an inventory list of staple items and restock regularly to prevent running out of essential ingredients.

Meal Prep and Storage Solutions

Meal prepping can be a lifesaver for busy families maintaining a GFCF diet. Preparing meals and snacks ahead of time ensures that safe, nutritious options are always available.

1. Batch Cooking

Choose one day of the week to batch-cook GFCF meals such as soups, stews, and casseroles. Portion these meals into individual containers and freeze them for easy grab-and-go options during the week.

2. Freezer-Friendly Staples

Stock your freezer with pre-prepared GFCF bread, muffins, and pancakes. This allows for quick breakfast or snack options without the need for daily cooking.

3. Storage Tips

Store GFCF foods in airtight containers to keep them fresh and prevent contamination. Use separate containers for GFCF foods and clearly label them to avoid confusion.

Label Reading 101

Learning to read labels effectively is crucial for avoiding hidden sources of gluten and casein. Here's a step-by-step guide to understanding what to look for on food packaging:

1.Scan for Allergen Warnings

Many food labels will list allergens such as wheat or milk. If a label states "Contains: Wheat" or "Contains: Milk," avoid that product.

2. Look for Certified GFCF Labels

Products labeled "Certified Gluten-Free" or "Dairy-Free" are the safest options. These labels indicate that the product has been tested to meet strict GFCF standards.

3. Identify Hidden Ingredients

Be cautious of ingredients like malt, modified food starch (unless specified as gluten-free), whey, and caseinates, which may not be immediately recognizable as sources of gluten or dairy.

4. Know the Safe Alternatives

Familiarize yourself with safe alternatives, such as using nutritional yeast instead of cheese for a savory flavor or arrowroot powder as a thickener instead of flour.

Tools and Gadgets for GFCF Cooking

The right tools can make GFCF meal preparation more efficient and enjoyable. Here are some recommended gadgets and equipment for a GFCF kitchen:

1. High-Speed Blender

A high-speed blender is perfect for making dairy-free smoothies, soups, and homemade GFCF ice cream.

2. Food Processor

Use a food processor for making hummus, seed bars, and finely chopping vegetables for meal prep.

3. Bread Machine with a Gluten-Free Setting

A bread machine with a gluten-free option can save time and effort when making homemade GFCF bread.

4. Spiralizer

A spiralizer is great for creating vegetable noodles from zucchini, sweet potatoes, or carrots as a pasta alternative.

5. Dedicated Toaster

Having a toaster that is only used for GFCF bread prevents cross-contamination and ensures a safe meal.

Creating a GFCF-Friendly Kitchen and Home Environment

1. Kitchen Setup Diagram

- Description: This diagram would depict a standard kitchen layout, with labeled sections for GFCF-only areas. Arrows and labels would indicate separate zones for storing GFCF foods, dedicated shelves for flours and grains, and specific drawers or containers for utensils and cookware used exclusively for GFCF meal prep.

- Key Features: Highlight dedicated cutting boards, color-coded utensils, separate toasters, and storage containers to prevent cross-contamination.

2. GFCF Pantry Layout

- Description: A visual of an organized pantry showing different sections labeled for essential GFCF items. This could include a shelf for baking supplies (gluten-free flours, baking powder), a section for grains (quinoa, rice, gluten-free oats), and jars for seeds and nuts.

- Key Features: Color-coded or labeled containers for easy identification, airtight jars for storage, and a checklist of must-have items.

3. Label Reading Guide

- Description: A sample food label illustration with highlighted areas showing where to look for "gluten-free" or "dairy-free" indications, allergen warnings, and common hidden ingredients like "malt" or "whey."

- Key Features: Annotations with arrows pointing out critical parts of the label, such as the ingredient list and allergen statement, with a brief explanation of what to avoid.

4. Meal Prep Workflow Chart

- Description: A step-by-step flowchart that guides readers through the meal prep process. Start with "Plan GFCF Meals," move to "Prepare Ingredients," followed by "Cook and Portion Meals," and end with "Store in Containers."

- Key Features: Icons for each step, such as a checklist for planning, a chopping board for preparing ingredients, a pot for cooking, and a labeled container for storage.

CHAPTER 16: The Emotional and Social Impact of a GFCF Lifestyle

Dietary restrictions can extend beyond the food on the table; they also impact emotional well-being and social interactions. Children and young adults who follow a GFCF diet may face challenges related to feeling different or excluded. This chapter explores how to navigate the emotional and social aspects of a lifestyle like this and offers strategies for fostering a positive relationship with food, building resilience, and creating inclusive social experiences.

When your child shares their feelings, it is important to practice active listening by responding with empathy rather than immediately offering solutions. This helps them feel heard and understood, validating their emotions. Encouraging younger children to express themselves through activities such as drawing or writing can also be beneficial, as it helps them articulate how they feel about their diet in a non-verbal way.

Local community centers and online platforms often host workshops where children can practice explaining their dietary needs. Participating in these workshops with other children who have similar experiences can boost their confidence. Role-playing different scenarios can further build social confidence. For example, you can practice how your child might explain their dietary needs to a friend's parent during a sleepover or ask about available snacks. Teaching them how to navigate school cafeteria situations by asking questions like, "What ingredients are in this dish?" or "Is this gluten-free?" equips them to handle real-life scenarios with more ease.

Helping your child build confidence through daily affirmations can reinforce positive thinking. Encouraging them to repeat phrases like, "I am confident in my food choices," or, "I can enjoy eating with my friends," can help boost their self-esteem. Another effective practice is engaging in mock interviews where your child practices ordering food at a restaurant in a playful and supportive setup. This makes the experience less intimidating and prepares them for similar situations in public.

Hosting inclusive events at home can help foster positive social experiences. Throwing a themed party where all the food is GFCF shows your child and their friends that safe food can be enjoyable for everyone. Planning a fun menu with GFCF pizza, cupcakes, and snacks can make the event more exciting. Sharing recipe cards with friends or their parents offers them an opportunity to learn how to make GFCF dishes that your child can safely eat. Cooking demonstrations are another great way to invite friends over and engage them in making simple GFCF recipes together. This turns meal prep into a shared, enjoyable activity and helps peers understand your child's dietary needs.

For managing anxiety and frustration, therapeutic activities such as guided relaxation can be effective. Teaching your child how to use guided relaxation apps or simple breathing techniques can help them stay calm during stressful food-related situations. Journaling can also provide an outlet for them to process emotions, with prompts like, "What went well today with my meals?" or, "How did I feel when explaining my diet to someone?" encouraging them to reflect on their experiences.

Creating support system worksheets can help your child identify people they can rely on for help and comfort. These worksheets might include sections such as "People I can talk to at school," "Friends who understand my diet," and "Family members who help me feel safe." This exercise reinforces that they are not alone and can lean on others for support.

Long-term coping strategies are essential for building resilience. Teaching your child that setbacks, such as accidentally consuming non-GFCF foods, are part of life and learning helps them understand that perfection isn't the goal. Reinforce the idea that growth comes from these moments. Encourage your child to practice mindfulness to manage anxiety around food situations. Simple practices such as focusing on their breathing or visualizing positive outcomes can be powerful tools for maintaining calm and confidence.

Family check-ins can be a great way to maintain communication and show ongoing support. Schedule weekly conversations to discuss how the GFCF diet is going, address what is working well, talk through challenges, and explore any improvements that could be made. Including siblings in these discussions and teaching them about the GFCF diet can help create an environment of empathy and shared responsibility. Siblings can be involved in cooking meals or learning about the risks of cross-contamination, making them active participants in the support system.

As a family, it's important to embrace flexibility. Dietary needs and preferences can change over time, and it's okay to make adjustments as new products become available or as your child's tastes evolve. When challenges arise, approach them with empathy, showing your child that they are supported no matter what. This compassionate approach reinforces that they are valued and understood, which helps build the confidence and resilience they need to thrive on a GFCF diet.

Understanding Emotional Challenges

Maintaining a GFCF diet can sometimes be emotionally taxing, particularly for children who are trying to fit in with their peers. Feelings of exclusion can arise when they find themselves unable to eat the same foods as their friends at parties, school events, or family gatherings. These moments can be difficult, and acknowledging your child's emotions is crucial for their mental and emotional well-being.

Creating an environment where your child feels comfortable sharing their feelings is essential. Encourage open communication by letting them express any frustrations or sadness about their diet. Listening with empathy, without judgment, helps them feel heard and supported. This validation allows your child to process these emotions and feel more secure in their dietary choices.

One helpful way to manage these emotions is by reframing the experience. Instead of focusing on the foods they can't have, emphasize the positives of their GFCF diet. Talk about how the foods they eat make them feel healthier, more energetic, and stronger. Focusing on the benefits—such as better digestion, improved focus, or feeling more energized—can help shift their perspective and make the diet feel like an empowering choice rather than a limitation.

Building Social Confidence

Building social confidence is an essential part of maintaining a GFCF lifestyle, especially when it comes to explaining dietary needs to friends, family, or classmates. Equip your child with the tools they need to confidently navigate social events where food might be a concern. This involves teaching them how to politely explain their dietary restrictions when necessary.

Role-playing social situations can be a great way to practice these conversations. Help your child rehearse simple phrases like, "I can't eat gluten or dairy because it makes me feel unwell," so that when they encounter similar scenarios, they feel prepared. Over time, this practice will help them feel more comfortable and confident in their ability to advocate for themselves.

Encourage your child to take ownership of their dietary choices by teaching them self-advocacy skills. This includes asking about food ingredients or preparation methods when dining out or visiting friends' houses. The more they practice these skills, the more confident they will become in maintaining their diet independently and handling social situations with ease.

Creating Inclusive Social Experiences

Ensuring your child feels included during social events can go a long way in improving their overall happiness and willingness to stick to their diet. One effective strategy is to bring GFCF-friendly dishes to social gatherings like parties or family events. By contributing a dish that everyone can enjoy, your child will have something to eat and will feel part of the group, rather than isolated because of their dietary restrictions.

Another way to ensure inclusivity is to host GFCF-friendly events at your own home. Plan playdates or parties where the entire menu is GFCF, making it easy for your child to enjoy the food without worrying about potential allergens. This approach not only supports your child's dietary needs but also helps educate their friends about how enjoyable GFCF foods can be.

Creating these inclusive experiences teaches your child that they do not have to sacrifice socializing or the joy of shared meals due to their dietary restrictions. It also provides an opportunity to normalize GFCF foods for others, helping to eliminate any stigma or discomfort associated with the diet.

Managing Anxiety and Frustration

Children who follow a GFCF diet may sometimes feel anxious or frustrated, particularly when they feel left out during social activities or meals. These feelings are completely normal, and supporting them emotionally is just as important as managing their diet itself.

Teaching your child simple mindfulness techniques can be incredibly helpful in managing stress and frustration. Practices like deep breathing, visualization, or even journaling can give your child healthy ways to process their emotions. For example, teaching your child the "4-7-8" breathing exercise—inhale for 4 counts, hold for 7 counts, and exhale for 8 counts—can help calm anxiety during challenging moments.

Additionally, celebrate your child's successes in adhering to their diet. Whether it's making healthy food choices at a social event or trying a new GFCF recipe at home, positive reinforcement can encourage your child to continue embracing their dietary choices with confidence and resilience. Acknowledging their efforts and progress helps build self-esteem and motivates them to stay committed to their health.

Parent and Family Support

A supportive family environment is crucial for helping a child maintain a GFCF diet, especially when they are still learning to navigate the challenges that come with it. When everyone in the family is on board and participating, your child will feel less isolated and more supported.

Involve the whole family in meal planning and preparation. When siblings and other family members are included in the process, it not only makes meal planning easier but also reinforces the idea that maintaining the diet is a collective effort, not just a responsibility for one person. This sense of unity can help reduce any feelings of frustration or resentment about dietary restrictions.

Parents also play an important role by leading by example. Embrace the GFCF lifestyle and model a positive attitude toward food. Show your child how to handle challenges with grace and how to approach difficult situations with a problem-solving mindset. When children see their parents navigating the diet with understanding and confidence, it teaches them how to adopt a similar mindset, making them more resilient and capable of dealing with challenges as they arise.

Final Thoughts

Understanding and managing the emotional and social aspects of a GFCF lifestyle are essential for ensuring long-term adherence and well-being. By equipping your child with the skills to handle social situations, supporting them emotionally, and fostering a positive home environment, you can help them thrive on a GFCF diet.

This holistic approach goes beyond food. It fosters emotional resilience, builds social confidence, and strengthens the sense of community. With the right support, your child can not only manage their diet but also embrace it as part of their identity, all while maintaining strong, healthy relationships with food and others.

The effort you put into addressing these emotional challenges will pay off, giving your child the tools they need to navigate the world with confidence, independence, and a sense of belonging.

CHAPTER 17 : Adapting the GFCF Diet to Arabic and Indian Cooking Cultures

The GFCF diet is primarily a Western concept, but as more people from diverse cultural backgrounds are adopting this dietary approach, the question of how to adapt traditional ethnic cuisines to be gluten- and dairy-free becomes increasingly important. This chapter focuses on how the GFCF diet aligns with Arabic and Indian cooking traditions, offering insight into how to modify staple recipes, travel tips, and ideas for maintaining cultural integrity while following a GFCF lifestyle.

Adapting GFCF to Arabic Cuisine

Arabic cuisine is known for its bold spices, fresh ingredients, and diverse range of dishes that often incorporate rice, lamb, chicken, vegetables, and legumes. Many dishes in Arabic cooking are naturally gluten-free and dairy-free, but there are several key areas where substitutions may be needed.

Naturally GFCF Dishes in Arabic Cooking

A significant portion of traditional Arabic meals is already compatible with the GFCF diet. These include:

1. Grilled meats and vegetables: Kabobs, shawarma, and grilled fish are typically made without gluten or dairy. Ensure that any marinades or seasonings do not contain hidden gluten, such as in soy sauce or pre-packaged spice mixes.

2. Hummus: This classic Middle Eastern dip made from chickpeas, tahini, olive oil, lemon, and garlic is naturally dairy-free and gluten-free. It's a nutritious and versatile food for snacks or meals.

3. Salads: Arabic salads like tabbouleh (made with parsley, tomatoes, onions, and lemon) and fattoush (cucumber, tomato, and lettuce salad with a lemon dressing) are naturally GFCF.

4. Rice-based dishes: Arabic pilafs such as maqluba (rice with vegetables and meat) or rice with lentils are typically made without gluten or dairy. Ensure the cooking process does not include butter or cream.

5. Vegetable stews: Dishes such as moussaka (eggplant stew) or loubieh (green beans in tomato sauce) are also safe, provided they are cooked without dairy or gluten-based thickeners.

Key Modifications for Arabic Cooking

While many Arabic dishes are naturally GFCF, several ingredients need to be substituted:

1. Bread: Arabic bread (like pita) is traditionally made with wheat flour. For a GFCF version, you can substitute with gluten-free flour or use store-bought gluten-free pita bread.

2. Dairy-based products: Yogurt and cheese (like labneh or feta) are commonly used in Arabic cuisine. These can be replaced with dairy-free yogurt or cheese alternatives made from cashews, almonds, or coconut.

3. Tahini: While tahini is typically dairy-free, always check the label to ensure there's no cross-contamination with gluten, especially if it's processed in a facility that handles gluten products.

4. Sweets: Arabic sweets such as baklava often contain butter and gluten-based phyllo dough. For a GFCF version, you can make it with gluten-free dough and use dairy-free margarine or coconut oil as a substitute for butter.

Arabic Cuisine on the Go: Traveling and Dining Out

Arabic cuisine is abundant in street food, but when traveling, you'll need to plan ahead:

- Street Food: Popular street foods like falafel (made from chickpeas) are naturally gluten-free. Just be cautious about where they are fried to avoid cross-contamination with gluten-containing foods.

- Restaurants: Many Arabic restaurants offer grilled meats, rice dishes, and vegetables. When dining out, ask the server about how food is prepared and whether any dairy or gluten-containing ingredients are added to the marinades, salads, or dips.

- Traveling in Arabic-speaking countries: In many parts of the Middle East and North Africa, traditional foods tend to be naturally free from gluten and dairy, but fast food and pre-packaged goods may contain hidden sources of gluten or casein. Learn the local terms for "gluten-free" and "dairy-free" in Arabic to help communicate dietary restrictions.

Adapting GFCF to Indian Cuisine

Indian cuisine is renowned for its vibrant spices, legumes, rice, and diverse flavors. Similar to Arabic cuisine, many Indian dishes are naturally gluten-free and dairy-free, but there are some key ingredients and cooking techniques to watch out for.

Naturally GFCF Dishes in Indian Cooking

Many Indian dishes can be enjoyed on a GFCF diet, as they use rice, vegetables, legumes, and various meats as staples. Some examples include:

- Rice dishes: Popular Indian rice dishes such as biryani, pulao, and khichdi (a rice and lentil dish) are often made without gluten or dairy. Just make sure that ghee (clarified butter) is substituted with plant-based oils such as coconut oil or olive oil.

- Lentil-based dishes: Dishes like dal (lentil stew) are naturally GFCF. These are rich in protein and can be made without dairy.

- Curries: Many curries, such as chana masala (chickpea curry), aloo gobi (potato and cauliflower curry), and palak paneer (spinach and cheese), can be adapted by swapping dairy for coconut milk or other plant-based options. However, be cautious with paneer (Indian cheese) as it contains casein.

- Vegetable dishes: Indian cuisine includes a wide array of vegetable dishes like baingan bharta (eggplant curry), aloo matar (potato and peas curry), and gobhi masala (cauliflower curry), which can be enjoyed without dairy or gluten.

Key Modifications for Indian Cooking

While many Indian dishes are naturally GFCF, there are several modifications to be aware of:

- Flour: Traditional Indian breads like naan, roti, and paratha are typically made with wheat flour. For GFCF versions, use gluten-free flours such as rice flour, chickpea flour, or a blend of gluten-free flours.

- Dairy: Dairy is widely used in Indian cooking, particularly in the form of yogurt, cream, and ghee. Substitute with dairy-free yogurt (coconut or almond-based) and replace ghee with plant-based oils such as olive oil, coconut oil, or vegan butters.

- Spices and ingredients: Many Indian spices such as cumin, coriander, turmeric, and garam masala are naturally GFCF. However, some pre-packaged spice mixes may contain additives, so it's important to check the label.

Indian Cuisine on the Go: Traveling and Dining Out

- Street Food: Street food is a large part of Indian culinary culture, with

items like samosas, pani puri, and pakoras commonly enjoyed. However, many of these are made with gluten and fried in oils that may also be used for gluten-based items. If you're traveling in India, look for places that specialize in vegetarian or vegan food, where you can more easily request gluten- and dairy-free options.

- Restaurants: When dining out in Indian restaurants, it's important to clarify which dishes are made with dairy or gluten. Indian restaurants typically offer a wide variety of vegetarian dishes, many of which are naturally GFCF. You can ask for modifications, such as replacing ghee with oil and avoiding cream-based curries.

- Traveling in India: Indian cuisine varies greatly by region, so it's useful to know the local food customs. For example, in South India, rice and lentils are staples, and many dishes are made with coconut milk, making them naturally dairy-free. In contrast, Northern Indian cuisine often includes dairy-heavy dishes, so it's important to ensure you're aware of substitutions.

GFCF Cooking While Traveling in Arabic and Indian Regions
When traveling to Arabic-speaking or Indian countries, there are a few key tips for managing a GFCF diet:

1. Learn Key Terms: Learning a few key terms in the local language can help in restaurants or markets. For example, in Arabic, "khalis" (خالص) means "pure" or "without" and can help when asking about foods containing gluten or dairy. Similarly, in Hindi or Urdu, you might use "bina doodh" (बिना दूध) for "without milk."

2. Pack Snacks: While local cuisine in many parts of the Middle East and India offers GFCF options, it's always wise to pack snacks. Gluten-free granola bars, dried fruits, or nuts can come in handy for long trips or when you're unsure about local options.

3. Research Restaurants: Many major cities in Arabic and Indian regions now have restaurants catering to dietary needs, including GFCF. Research ahead of time or use apps like HappyCow to find allergy-friendly dining spots.

4. Stay Flexible: While traditional foods from Arabic and Indian cuisines may often be GFCF, fast food and pre-packaged meals may contain gluten or dairy. Always be vigilant about cross-contamination and ask about food preparation methods.

Chapter: Adapting the GFCF Diet to Chinese Cuisine

Chinese cuisine is incredibly diverse, offering a wide range of flavors, ingredients, and cooking methods. It has a rich history of balancing savory, sweet, sour, and umami tastes, often incorporating vegetables, rice, noodles, seafood, and meats. Like many other global cuisines, Chinese food can be adapted to meet the requirements of a GFCF diet, but careful attention to ingredients and cooking methods is essential. This chapter will explore how to adapt Chinese food for a GFCF lifestyle, whether cooking at home, dining out, or traveling

Naturally GFCF Dishes in Chinese Cooking

Many Chinese dishes are naturally gluten-free and dairy-free, particularly those based on fresh ingredients, rice, vegetables, and meats. Here are a few examples of naturally GFCF dishes you can enjoy:

- Steamed Dishes: Chinese steamed fish or chicken dishes are often GFCF, as they rely on fresh proteins and simple seasoning. Ensure that the seasonings used, like soy sauce, are gluten-free or replaced with alternatives like tamari or coconut aminos.

- Stir-Fried Vegetables: Stir-frying is a staple of Chinese cooking, and many vegetable dishes are naturally GFCF. Dishes like stir-fried bok choy, Chinese broccoli (gai lan), and eggplant with garlic can be easily adapted to the GFCF diet.

- Congee: This rice porridge dish, often served with meats or vegetables, can be GFCF if made with a simple broth and no dairy or gluten additives.

- Rice and Noodles: Traditional Chinese rice-based dishes such as fried rice and steamed rice are usually GFCF. You can also substitute gluten-containing noodles with rice noodles or other gluten-free options for dishes like pad thai or pho (if you're seeking an inspired Chinese noodle dish).

Modifications for Common Chinese Dishes

While many Chinese dishes are naturally GFCF, some require modifications due to the use of gluten and dairy products in traditional recipes:

- Soy Sauce: Traditional soy sauce contains wheat, making it unsuitable for a GFCF diet. However, there are excellent alternatives, such as tamari (which is often gluten-free), coconut aminos, or Bragg Liquid Aminos. These alternatives offer a similar flavor profile without the gluten.

- Dumplings: Chinese dumplings are typically made with wheat flour and filled with meats, vegetables, or tofu. To make them GFCF, you can substitute the dough with gluten-free flour or rice flour-based wrappers. Similarly, you can use coconut milk or vegetable broth instead of traditional stock for added flavor.

- Noodles: Many traditional Chinese noodles are made with wheat. However, there are gluten-free noodle options, such as rice noodles (used in dishes like chow fun) or sweet potato noodles, which can be easily substituted in most recipes.

- Broths and Sauces: Many Chinese broths and sauces contain hidden gluten, such as in pre-made stocks or seasoning packets. Always read the labels carefully or make broths from scratch using vegetable, chicken, or beef bases, ensuring no gluten-containing ingredients are used.

GFCF Ingredients Commonly Used in Chinese Cooking
Here's a list of ingredients that are either naturally gluten-free or can be substituted to make your Chinese cooking GFCF:

- Rice: Whether you're using white rice, jasmine rice, or brown rice, rice is a staple of Chinese cuisine and is naturally gluten-free.

- Rice Noodles: Used in dishes like pad thai, chow mein, and pho, rice noodles are a fantastic GFCF alternative to wheat-based noodles.

- Tofu: Tofu is naturally dairy- and gluten-free, making it a great protein option in stir-fries, soups, and hot pots. Just be cautious with pre-marinated tofu, as it may contain gluten or dairy.

- Tamari and Coconut Aminos: Both are excellent replacements for soy sauce and can be used in any recipe that requires soy sauce.

- Cornstarch: Often used as a thickening agent in Chinese cooking, cornstarch is gluten-free and can replace flour-based thickeners.

- Ginger and Garlic: These foundational flavors in Chinese cuisine are naturally gluten-free and dairy-free, adding rich depth to dishes.

- Sesame Oil: A common cooking oil used in Chinese dishes, sesame oil is typically gluten-free and dairy-free.

Chinese Food on the Go: Traveling and Dining Out

Traveling and dining out in Chinese restaurants while maintaining a GFCF diet can be challenging due to the widespread use of soy sauce, wheat-based noodles, and hidden gluten or dairy in sauces. However, with a few adjustments and strategies, it is entirely possible to enjoy Chinese food while traveling or dining out.

Dining in Chinese Restaurants

When dining at a Chinese restaurant, communication is key. Here are some tips for navigating Chinese menus:

- Ask for GFCF Alternatives: Many Chinese restaurants are familiar with dietary restrictions. Don't hesitate to ask the server if they offer tamari or coconut aminos as substitutes for soy sauce. If you're ordering stir-fries or soups, ask them to hold any wheat-based ingredients or dairy.

- Go for Simple Dishes: Opt for simple, rice-based dishes or stir-fried vegetables, which are often naturally GFCF. Be cautious with pre-made sauces or condiments that may contain gluten or dairy.

- Avoid Thickened Sauces: Some sauces may be thickened with flour, so it's best to request sauces on the side or ask for a substitute. Cornstarch is typically used for thickening in GFCF dishes.

- Clarify the Use of Broth: Many Chinese dishes, especially soups, are made with broth that may contain gluten or dairy. It's important to clarify whether the broth is GFCF and to ask for alternative broth options, like vegetable broth, if necessary.

Traveling in China or Chinese-speaking Regions

When traveling in China or other regions with large Chinese-speaking populations, maintaining a GFCF diet can be more challenging due to the prevalence of soy sauce and gluten-rich dishes. However, there are ways to manage:

- Learn Key Phrases: Learning a few essential phrases in Mandarin, Cantonese, or the local dialect can be helpful when communicating dietary restrictions. For example, in Mandarin, you can say, "**我不吃面筋和奶制品**" (wǒ bù chī miàn jīn hé nǎi zhì pǐn), which means "I don't eat gluten and dairy."

- Street Food: Traditional street food like dumplings, baozi (steamed buns), and jianbing (savory pancakes) often contains gluten and dairy, so it's important to ask about the ingredients or avoid them altogether. Instead, try grilled meats, rice, or vegetable-based dishes that are more likely to be GFCF.

- Grocery Stores: If you're staying in China for an extended period, consider shopping at grocery stores that sell rice noodles, rice, tofu, and vegetables. Many larger cities have international supermarkets or local markets where you can find GFCF-friendly ingredients.

Modifying Chinese Recipes for GFCF

Here are a few popular Chinese recipes and tips for making them GFCF:

- Sweet and Sour Chicken: Traditional sweet and sour chicken is often battered and fried with gluten. For a GFCF version, use rice flour for the batter, and replace any soy sauce with tamari or coconut aminos. The sauce can be thickened with cornstarch, and use apple cider vinegar or rice vinegar for the tangy flavor.

- Chow Mein: Substitute traditional wheat noodles with rice noodles and ensure that the stir-fry sauce is made with tamari or coconut aminos. Add vegetables like bell peppers, carrots, and broccoli for a balanced dish.

- Kung Pao Chicken: This flavorful stir-fry can be made GFCF by using tamari instead of soy sauce, and ensuring that no gluten-containing ingredients are used for the sauce. Substitute cornstarch for any flour-based thickening agents.

- Hot and Sour Soup: Replace any gluten-based broth with a GFCF alternative (like vegetable broth), and ensure that the soup's seasoning mix is free from gluten. The thickening agent should be cornstarch.

Final Thoughts

Adapting the GFCF diet to Arabic and Indian cuisines involves a mix of understanding traditional foods, making smart substitutions, and becoming familiar with local ingredients. By recognizing which dishes are naturally compatible and learning how to modify others, you can enjoy rich, flavorful meals without compromising your dietary needs. Whether you're cooking at home, dining out, or traveling, maintaining a GFCF lifestyle while honoring cultural traditions can be both practical and rewarding.

This chapter has provided an overview of how to make Arabic and Indian cuisines GFCF-friendly, offering practical tips for substitutions, dining out, and traveling. By making a few adjustments and being mindful of ingredients, it's entirely possible to enjoy these rich culinary traditions while maintaining a healthy, gluten-free, and casein-free lifestyle.

Adapting the GFCF diet to Chinese cuisine requires awareness of certain ingredients and the ability to make smart substitutions. With a little knowledge and flexibility, it's possible to enjoy a wide variety of Chinese dishes without compromising your dietary needs. Whether you're cooking at home, dining out, or traveling, Chinese cuisine can still be part of a GFCF lifestyle by simply avoiding gluten and dairy-rich components and using thoughtful alternatives.

This chapter has provided practical advice on how to modify Chinese recipes, tips for dining out, and suggestions for traveling in Chinese-speaking regions while maintaining a GFCF diet. By making these adjustments, you can continue to enjoy the flavors of Chinese cuisine while adhering to the GFCF lifestyle.

RECIPES: Delicious GFCF Recipes for Every Occasion

Creating a comprehensive set of GFCF recipes helps ensure that your child enjoys a variety of tasty, safe meals and snacks. This section includes recipes for birthday cakes, cookies, pancakes, bagels, bread, smoothies, hummus, and more, so you have options for everyday meals, snacks, and special occasions.

GFCF Birthday Cake Recipe

Ingredients:

2 ½ cups gluten-free all-purpose flour

1 ½ cups coconut sugar or granulated sugar

1 tbsp baking powder

½ tsp baking soda

1 tsp salt

1 cup dairy-free milk (such as almond or oat milk)

½ cup melted coconut oil or dairy-free butter

3 large eggs or egg replacer

1 tbsp vanilla extract

½ cup warm water

Instructions:

1.Preheat the oven to 350°F (175°C). Grease and line two 8-inch round cake pans with parchment paper.

2.In a large bowl, mix the gluten-free flour, sugar, baking powder, baking soda, and salt.

3.Add the dairy-free milk, melted coconut oil, eggs, and vanilla extract. Mix until well combined.

4.Gradually add the warm water and continue mixing until the batter is smooth.

5.Divide the batter between the prepared pans and smooth the tops.

6.Bake for 25-30 minutes or until a toothpick inserted in the center comes out clean.

7.Let the cakes cool in the pans for 10 minutes before transferring to a wire rack to cool completely.

8.Frost with dairy-free frosting and decorate as desired.

GFCF Cookies Recipe

Ingredients:

1 ½ cups gluten-free all-purpose flour

½ cup coconut sugar or brown sugar

½ tsp baking soda

¼ tsp salt

½ cup dairy-free butter or coconut oil

1 egg or egg replacer

1 tsp vanilla extract

½ cup dairy-free chocolate chips

Instructions:

1.Preheat the oven to 350°F (175°C). Line a baking sheet with parchment paper.

2.Combine gluten-free flour, baking soda, and salt in a bowl.

3.In a separate bowl, cream dairy-free butter and sugar until smooth. Add the egg and vanilla extract and mix well.

4.Gradually mix the dry ingredients into the wet mixture and stir until combined.

5.Fold in the dairy-free chocolate chips.

6.Drop spoonfuls of dough onto the prepared baking sheet.

7.Bake for 8-10 minutes or until edges are golden brown.

8.Let cool on the baking sheet for 5 minutes before transferring to a wire rack.

GFCF Pancake Recipe
Ingredients:

1 ½ cups gluten-free all-purpose flour

1 tbsp coconut sugar or granulated sugar

1 tbsp baking powder

½ tsp salt

1 ¼ cups dairy-free milk

1 egg or egg replacer

3 tbsp melted coconut oil or dairy-free butter

1 tsp vanilla extract

Instructions:

1.In a large bowl, whisk together the gluten-free flour, sugar, baking powder, and salt.

2.Add the dairy-free milk, egg, melted coconut oil, and vanilla extract. Mix until just combined.

3.Heat a non-stick pan or griddle over medium heat. Pour ¼ cup of batter for each pancake.

4.Cook until bubbles form on the surface, then flip and cook for another 1-2 minutes.

5.Serve with GFCF syrup, fresh fruit, or dairy-free yogurt.

GFCF Bagels Recipe

Ingredients:

2 cups gluten-free all-purpose flour

2 ½ tsp baking powder

½ tsp salt

1 cup dairy-free Greek yogurt

1 egg (for egg wash)

Instructions:

1.Preheat the oven to 375°F (190°C). Line a baking sheet with parchment paper.

2.Combine the gluten-free flour, baking powder, and salt in a large bowl.

3.Add the dairy-free Greek yogurt and mix until a dough forms.

4.Divide the dough into 4-6 pieces and shape each piece into a bagel.

5.Brush each bagel with an egg wash.

6.Bake for 20-25 minutes or until golden brown.

7.Let cool before serving.

GFCF Bread Recipe
Ingredients:

3 cups gluten-free all-purpose flour

1 tbsp xanthan gum (omit if your flour mix already includes it)

2 ¼ tsp active dry yeast

1 ½ cups warm water

2 tbsp olive oil

2 tbsp honey or maple syrup

1 tsp salt

Instructions:

1.In a bowl, combine the yeast and warm water and let it sit for 5 minutes.

2.In a separate large bowl, mix the gluten-free flour, xanthan gum, and salt.

3.Add the olive oil and honey to the yeast mixture and stir.

4.Gradually mix the wet ingredients into the dry ingredients until a dough forms.

5.Transfer the dough to a greased loaf pan and let it rise in a warm place for 30-45 minutes.

6.Preheat the oven to 375°F (190°C).

7.Bake for 35-40 minutes or until the bread is golden brown and sounds hollow when tapped.

8.Cool completely before slicing.

GFCF Smoothie Recipe
Ingredients:

1 banana

1 cup frozen berries (strawberries, blueberries, or raspberries)

1 cup dairy-free milk

1 tbsp chia seeds or flaxseed

1 tbsp dairy-free yogurt (optional)

Honey or maple syrup to taste (optional)

Instructions:

1.Add all ingredients to a blender.

2.Blend until smooth and creamy.

3.Serve immediately for a refreshing, nutrient-packed drink.

GFCF Hummus Recipe

Ingredients:

1 can (15 oz) chickpeas, drained and rinsed

¼ cup tahini

2 tbsp olive oil

2 tbsp lemon juice

1 garlic clove, minced

½ tsp salt

Water as needed

Instructions:

1.Add the chickpeas, tahini, olive oil, lemon juice, garlic, and salt to a food processor.

2.Blend until smooth, adding water as needed to achieve the desired consistency.

3.Serve with gluten-free crackers or fresh vegetables.

GFCF Muffins Recipe

Ingredients:

2 cups gluten-free all-purpose flour

1 tbsp baking powder

½ tsp salt

½ cup coconut sugar or brown sugar

1 cup dairy-free milk

¼ cup melted coconut oil or dairy-free butter

2 eggs or egg replacers

1 tsp vanilla extract

Optional: ½ cup blueberries or dairy-free chocolate chips

Instructions:

1.Preheat the oven to 350°F (175°C). Line a muffin tin with paper liners.

2.Mix the flour, baking powder, salt, and sugar in a bowl.

3.In another bowl, combine the dairy-free milk, melted coconut oil, eggs, and vanilla extract.

4.Add the wet ingredients to the dry ingredients and mix until just combined.

5.Fold in the blueberries or chocolate chips if desired.

6.Fill the muffin liners about ⅔ full and bake for 20-25 minutes.

7.Let cool before serving.

GFCF Banana Bread Recipe

Ingredients:

2 cups gluten-free all-purpose flour

1 tsp baking soda

½ tsp salt

½ cup coconut sugar or granulated sugar

2-3 ripe bananas, mashed

½ cup melted coconut oil or dairy-free butter

2 eggs or egg replacers

1 tsp vanilla extract

Instructions:

1.Preheat the oven to 350°F (175°C). Grease a loaf pan.

2.Combine the flour, baking soda, salt, and sugar in a bowl.

3.In another bowl, mix the mashed bananas, melted coconut oil, eggs, and vanilla.

4.Add the wet ingredients to the dry ingredients and stir until combined.

5.Pour the batter into the loaf pan and bake for 50-60 minutes.

6.Cool in the pan for 10 minutes, then transfer to a wire rack.

This comprehensive collection of GFCF recipes provides a range of options for any occasion, ensuring that your child can enjoy delicious and safe foods, from special celebrations to daily meals and snacks.

GFCF Seed Bar Recipe

Ingredients:

1 cup sunflower seeds

½ cup pumpkin seeds

½ cup chia seeds

½ cup flaxseeds

1 cup shredded unsweetened coconut

½ cup honey or maple syrup

¼ cup melted coconut oil

1 tsp vanilla extract

A pinch of salt

Instructions:

1.Preheat the oven to 325°F (160°C). Line an 8x8-inch baking pan with parchment paper.

2.In a large bowl, combine sunflower seeds, pumpkin seeds, chia seeds, flaxseeds, shredded coconut, and salt.

3.In a small saucepan, gently heat the honey or maple syrup, melted coconut oil, and vanilla extract until well combined.

4.Pour the wet mixture over the seed mix and stir until everything is well coated.

5.Press the mixture firmly into the prepared pan.

6.Bake for 20-25 minutes or until golden brown.

7.Let cool completely before cutting into bars. Store in an airtight container.

GFCF Homemade Ice Cream Alternative

Ingredients:

2 cups dairy-free milk (coconut, almond, or oat milk)

½ cup dairy-free coconut cream (for creaminess)

½ cup maple syrup or honey

1 tbsp vanilla extract

Optional mix-ins: dairy-free chocolate chips, fruit, or nuts

Instructions:

1.In a blender, combine the dairy-free milk, coconut cream, maple syrup, and vanilla extract. Blend until smooth.

2.Pour the mixture into an ice cream maker and churn according to the manufacturer's instructions. If you don't have an ice cream maker, pour the mixture into a shallow dish, cover, and freeze. Stir every 30 minutes until it reaches your desired consistency (about 3-4 hours).

3.Fold in any optional mix-ins and freeze for another hour if needed.

4.Serve scoops topped with dairy-free chocolate chips or fresh fruit.

GFCF Ice Lollies Recipe

Ingredients:

2 cups dairy-free yogurt (coconut, almond, or soy yogurt)

1 cup mixed berries (strawberries, blueberries, raspberries)

2 tbsp honey or maple syrup

1 tsp lemon juice

Instructions:

1.In a blender, combine the dairy-free yogurt, berries, honey or maple syrup, and lemon juice. Blend until smooth.

2.Pour the mixture into ice lolly molds.

3.Insert sticks and freeze for at least 4-6 hours or until fully set.

4.Run warm water over the molds for a few seconds to help release the ice lollies before serving.

GFCF Energy Bites Recipe

Ingredients:

1 cup gluten-free rolled oats

½ cup peanut butter or almond butter

⅓ cup honey or maple syrup

¼ cup dairy-free chocolate chips

¼ cup chia seeds or flaxseed meal

1 tsp vanilla extract

Instructions:

1.In a bowl, combine all the ingredients until well-mixed.

2.Roll the mixture into small balls (about 1 inch in diameter).

3.Place the energy bites on a tray and refrigerate for at least 1 hour before serving.

4.Store in an airtight container in the fridge for up to a week.

GFCF Fruit Sorbet Recipe

Ingredients:

4 cups frozen mango chunks (or any preferred fruit)

½ cup dairy-free coconut water or juice

2 tbsp honey or maple syrup (optional)

Instructions:

1.Add the frozen mango chunks and coconut water to a food processor or high-speed blender.

2.Blend until smooth, stopping to scrape down the sides as needed. Add honey or maple syrup if you prefer a sweeter taste.

3.Transfer to an airtight container and freeze for 1-2 hours for a firmer texture.

4.Scoop and serve with fresh fruit on top.

GFCF Chocolate-Dipped Banana Pops

Ingredients:

3 bananas, peeled and cut in half crosswise

1 cup dairy-free chocolate chips

1 tbsp coconut oil

Chopped nuts, shredded coconut, or sprinkles for toppings

Instructions:

1.Insert popsicle sticks into the cut ends of the banana halves.

2.In a microwave-safe bowl, melt the dairy-free chocolate chips and coconut oil in 30-second intervals, stirring between each, until fully melted.

3.Dip each banana half into the melted chocolate, coating evenly.

4.Roll the chocolate-covered bananas in your choice of toppings.

5.Place on a parchment-lined baking sheet and freeze for at least 2 hours before serving.

GFCF Banana Mud Cake with Peanut Butter Caramel

Ingredients:

For the Cake:

100g vegetable shortening (ensure it's dairy-free)

30g cacao butter

140g banana puree (smooth, no chunks)

250ml plant-based milk (such as almond, oat, or coconut milk, unsweetened)

2 tablespoons white vinegar (to curdle the plant-based milk)

1 tablespoon vanilla extract

100ml boiling water

270g gluten-free all-purpose flour (ensure it's a blend without wheat)

30g cornflour (cornstarch)

208g caster sugar (or a suitable sugar substitute)

1½ teaspoons baking powder (ensure it's gluten-free)

½ teaspoon salt

For the Peanut Butter Caramel Filling:

200g caster sugar (or a suitable sugar substitute)

60ml water

1 tablespoon white vinegar

100g thick coconut cream (use full-fat coconut milk as a substitute)

65g natural crunchy peanut butter (check for no added dairy or sugar)

Instructions:

1.Prepare the Cake:

- Preheat the oven to 150°C (302°F). Line two 6-inch (15.24 cm) cake tins with baking paper, grease with oil, and dust with gluten-free flour.

- Melt the vegetable shortening and cacao butter in a small pot over low heat. Once melted, remove from heat and whisk in the banana puree until combined.

- In a separate jug, mix the plant-based milk with white vinegar and allow it to curdle for a minute or two, then add the vanilla extract and whisk until smooth.

- In the bowl of a stand mixer or large mixing bowl, sift together the gluten-free flour, cornflour, caster sugar, baking powder, and salt. Mix on low speed until evenly combined.

- Slowly add the banana mixture to the dry ingredients, mixing on the lowest speed until just combined. Scrape down the sides of the bowl, then mix for a few more seconds.

- Gradually pour in the boiling water along the side of the bowl, mixing on the lowest speed. Once incorporated, scrape down the sides and mix again on low for a few seconds.

- Divide the batter evenly between the prepared tins, tap the tins on the bench to release air bubbles, and bake for 43-45 minutes. Check with a skewer through the center; if it comes out clean, the cake is ready.

- Allow the cakes to cool in the tins for 10 minutes, then transfer to a wire rack to cool completely.

2.Prepare the Peanut Butter Caramel Filling:

- Combine the caster sugar and water in a saucepan. Stir over low heat until the sugar dissolves completely. Once dissolved, increase the heat to high and bring to a boil without stirring. Allow it to boil until it reaches a golden caramel color, being careful not to burn it.

- Remove from heat and let it sit for a minute. Slowly stir in the coconut cream (it will bubble, so do it gently) until fully combined. Return to medium heat and boil for a minute while stirring.

- Stir in the peanut butter until smooth and fully incorporated. Allow the caramel to cool and thicken. If it becomes too thick, gently warm it again and stir in more coconut cream to adjust the consistency.

3.Assemble the Cake:

- Once the cakes have cooled, place one layer on a serving plate. Spread a generous amount of the peanut butter caramel filling over the top.

- Place the second cake layer on top and press down gently to adhere.

- Optionally, you can frost the top and sides of the cake with extra peanut butter caramel or your favorite GFCF frosting.

GFCF Banana Pancakes

A simple and tasty breakfast or snack option.

Ingredients:

2 ripe bananas

2 eggs

1/2 tsp baking powder (ensure it's gluten-free)

1/2 tsp vanilla extract

1/4 tsp cinnamon

A pinch of salt

Coconut oil (for frying)

Instructions:

1.Mash the bananas in a bowl until smooth.

2.In another bowl, whisk the eggs and then add the mashed bananas, baking powder, vanilla, cinnamon, and salt. Mix well.

3.Heat coconut oil in a pan over medium heat.

4.Pour small scoops of the pancake mixture into the pan and cook for 2-3 minutes on each side or until golden brown.

5.Serve with maple syrup, fresh berries, or a sprinkle of powdered sugar.

GFCF Sweet Potato Fries

A nutritious and crispy side dish or snack.

Ingredients:

2 large sweet potatoes

2 tbsp olive oil

1/2 tsp paprika

1/4 tsp garlic powder

Salt and pepper to taste

Instructions:

1.Preheat oven to 425°F (220°C). Line a baking sheet with parchment paper.

2.Peel the sweet potatoes and cut them into fries.

3.Toss the fries with olive oil, paprika, garlic powder, salt, and pepper.

4.Spread the fries in a single layer on the baking sheet.

5.Bake for 25-30 minutes, flipping halfway through, until crispy and golden.

6.Serve with a GFCF-friendly dipping sauce, such as ketchup or guacamole.

GFCF *Avocado Chocolate Mousse*

A creamy, rich dessert that's easy to make and completely dairy-free.

Ingredients:

2 ripe avocados

1/4 cup unsweetened cocoa powder

1/4 cup maple syrup

1 tsp vanilla extract

A pinch of salt

Dairy-free chocolate chips (optional for garnish)

Instructions:

1.In a blender or food processor, combine the avocados, cocoa powder, maple syrup, vanilla extract, and salt. Blend until smooth.

2.Taste and adjust the sweetness by adding more maple syrup if desired.

3.Spoon the mousse into small serving bowls and refrigerate for at least an hour before serving.

4.Top with dairy-free chocolate chips or fresh berries for extra flavor.

GFCF Zucchini Noodles with Pesto

A light, fresh meal or side dish that's full of flavor.

Ingredients:

2 zucchinis, spiralized into noodles

1/4 cup pine nuts (or sunflower seeds as an alternative)

1 cup fresh basil leaves

1/4 cup olive oil

2 tbsp nutritional yeast (optional, but adds a cheesy flavor)

1 garlic clove

Salt and pepper to taste

Instructions:

1.To make the pesto, blend the basil, pine nuts, olive oil, nutritional yeast, garlic, salt, and pepper in a food processor until smooth.

2.In a pan, heat a little olive oil over medium heat. Add the zucchini noodles and cook for 2-3 minutes, just until tender.

3.Toss the zucchini noodles with the pesto and serve immediately.

GFCF Apple Oatmeal Cookies

These cookies are gluten-free and dairy-free, with a delicious apple cinnamon flavor.

Ingredients:

2 ripe bananas, mashed

1 cup gluten-free rolled oats

1/2 cup unsweetened applesauce

1/4 tsp cinnamon

1/4 tsp vanilla extract

A pinch of salt

1/4 cup raisins (optional)

1/4 cup chopped nuts (optional)

Instructions:

1. Preheat the oven to 350°F (175°C). Line a baking sheet with parchment paper.

2. In a bowl, combine the mashed bananas, oats, applesauce, cinnamon, vanilla extract, and salt. Mix until fully combined.

3. Fold in raisins or nuts if desired.

4. Drop spoonfuls of the dough onto the prepared baking sheet, flattening them slightly.

5. Bake for 12-15 minutes, until the cookies are golden brown around the edges.

6. Let the cookies cool before serving.

GFCF Chickpea Salad

A light and refreshing salad, perfect as a side dish or a light meal.

Ingredients:

1 can (15 oz) chickpeas, drained and rinsed

1 cucumber, diced

1 red bell pepper, diced

1/2 red onion, finely chopped

1/4 cup fresh parsley, chopped

2 tbsp olive oil

1 tbsp lemon juice

Salt and pepper to taste

Instructions:

1.In a large bowl, combine the chickpeas, cucumber, bell pepper, onion, and parsley.

2.Drizzle with olive oil and lemon juice, then season with salt and pepper to taste.

3.Toss everything together and serve immediately. This salad can also be stored in the fridge for a few hours to allow the flavors to meld.

GFCF Mango Sorbet

A sweet, refreshing dessert that's easy to make with only a few ingredients.

Ingredients:

2 ripe mangoes, peeled and chopped

1/2 cup coconut water (or any other plant-based liquid)

1-2 tbsp honey or maple syrup (optional)

Instructions:

1.In a blender, combine the mango chunks, coconut water, and sweetener (if using).

2.Blend until smooth, adding more coconut water if needed to reach the desired consistency.

3.Pour the mixture into an airtight container and freeze for at least 4 hours or until frozen.

4. Scoop out the sorbet and serve in bowls.

These recipes offer a range of fun and healthy snack options, from protein-packed seed bars to refreshing ice lollies and indulgent chocolate-dipped banana pops. Your child will enjoy the variety of flavors and textures, making it easy to stick to a GFCF diet while savoring delicious treats.

REFERENCES

BDA https://www.bda.uk.com/resource/autism-diet.html

Elemy https://elemy.wpengine.com/autism-and-diet/food-list

National Autistic Society https://www.autism.org.uk/advice-and-guidance/topics/behaviour/eating/all-audiences

Neurolaunch https://neurolaunch.com/autism-diet/

Autism Research Institute https://autism.org/summary-diet-nutrition-medical-treatments

Nourishing Hope For Autism https://nourishing-hope.com/nourishing-hope-for-autism